MW00831294

THE WAVEFORM SYMBOL BOOK

A Description of the 33 Waveform Symbols

and Ways to Use the Waveform Deck

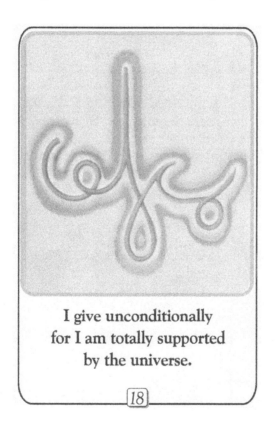

I give unconditionally
for I am totally supported
by the universe.

18

Artistic Rendering of the Symbols by Paul Bond

PUBLISHED BY NEW EARTH HORIZON
UNAUTHORIZED PHOTOCOPYING CREATES KARMA

A New Earth Horizon Publication
The waveform Symbol Book

PUBLISHED BY
New Earth Horizon
Pagosa Springs, Colorado USA

No part of this book may be reproduced or transmitted in any form
or by any means, electronic or mechanical, including photocopying,
recording, or by any information storage and retrieval system, without
permission in writing from the publisher.

ISBN 978-0-9847373-5-2

1. Body Mind & Spirit, 2. Health & Fitness, 3. Self Help, 4. Author, 5. Title

Library of Congress Cataloging-in-Publication Data is available upon
request.

Copyright © 2001-2013 by Samuel Welsh
Cover and copy art copyrighted © 2001-2013 by New Earth Horizon

All rights reserved
Printed in the United States of America

First Edition, June 15, 2013
10 9 8 7 6 5 4 3 2 1

Important Note

The energy balancing techniques discussed in this book are not suggested as a replacement for medical diagnosis and treatment. Contact your doctor if medical complications arise.

DEDICATION

This book is dedicated to the memory of Saint Francis of Assisi who demonstrated that one can transform suffering into lobe through the recognition of the presence of Source within oneself and within the world.

Also by Samuel Welsh

CREATING SACRED SPACES FOR COMMUNITIES

TRANSFORMING INNER STRESS:
THE POLARITY RESOLUTION PROCESS (P.R.P.)

THE MULTILEVEL BALANCING PROCESS

TABLE OF CONTENTS

A SHORT STORY ON THE WAVEFORM SYMBOLS

Entering the Cave of Symbols

In 1989 I attended an evening spiritual course. During one of the classes we practiced meditation. In this class I successfully meditated for the first time.

I was deep in meditation when in my mind's eye this vision unfolded. I stood at the base of an enormous and grand mountain. I could see a very small black dot near the top of the mountain face. I knew at that moment it was a mouth of a cave. I had a strong impulse to investigate the cave and with that choice I found myself instantly inside it.

Within the cave I saw symbols carved into the walls—thousands of symbols carved in gold light. A soft gold glow emanated from the symbols and infused the cave's interior.

The cave felt hallowed. I knew the sacred feeling arose because of the presence of the symbols. The cave also felt ancient as if it had been there since the beginning of time.

(Later, I was informed through a channel that such a cave exists in the future on another dimension and is called the *Cave of the Ancients*, belonging to the *Order of Melchizedeck*.)

When I related my vision to my course instructor, he became excited and suggested I attempt to return to the cave and to see whether I could replicate any of the symbols.

Accessing the Symbols

After many trials, I trained myself in meditation to return to the cave and access specific symbols. I would enter the *Cave of Symbols* (in meditation) with the intention to connect with a symbol for a specific quality, such as for *Divine Freedom* (Symbol #12).

Once I felt connected to the symbol's energy, I would begin to draw the symbol in the air. I discovered I could energetically feel the correct shape and form of the symbol kinesthetically.

It Is a Symbolic Language

After more than twenty years of accessing *Waveform Symbols* (over 500 of them), I now believe that the *Waveform Symbols* are a specific symbolic language used at a particular dimensional level of the universe. Any language has an alphabet of letters. We string the letters together to form words.

The symbolic letters in the Waveform language are smaller symbols such as a clockwise spiral, a counterclockwise spiral, a vertical infinity sign, a horizontal infinity sign, etc. These smaller symbolic letters are then connected together to form larger symbols, which are the symbolic words, each with their own unique combinational frequency.

(A psychic, upon seeing the card deck, said that all the *Waveform Symbols*—of which there are millions on a higher dimension—were the *Language of Enoch*.)

When you draw or paint the symbols, you start at the far left and move to the right in one fluid motion.

Waveform Symbol Holograms

I perceive any two-dimensional *Waveform Symbol* rather like a post office box key with which you can open a very large post office box and acquire a lot of information. The key does not hold the information that is contained in the post office box; it only allows you to retrieve the information in the box.

I believe the Waveform holographic information is higher dimensional in nature and the *Waveform Symbol*, through resonant frequency coupling, connects you with that higher dimensional hologram, allowing its energy and information to be easily accessed.

An intuitive friend upon looking at a *Waveform Symbol* saw a three-dimensional image of an energy field expanding, contracting, and spinning. He also saw it pulsating and scintillating in colors. I believe he was actually seeing the *Waveform Symbol's* hologram.

The Wave Aspect

Light has a dual nature, depending upon how you study it. It can express itself as either a particle (a photon) or as a probability wave moving upon and within the Universal energy field.

I believe these symbols work with the wave aspect of light. Eventually, I began calling the symbolic language "Waveform" to convey this notion.

My First Explorations with Symbol Cards

During 1990, I used the *Waveform Symbols* almost exclusively upon myself. I created a deck of hand-drawn *Waveform Symbols* on blank index cards with colored pens. I utilized the symbol card deck in the same manner as outlined in this book. That is, when an emotional issue came up, I would connect with my Higher Self and ask which symbols would help me clear the emotional charge.

After selecting the appropriate symbol cards, I would ask my Higher Self to assist in transferring their vibrational essence into my Being (see *Chapter 1*). I found this process so helpful and powerful, I used my symbol card deck daily for two years.

Using the Waveform Symbol Cards in Crystal Grids

In 1992, I began expanding the application of the *Waveform Symbols* and experimented with their use in crystal grids. I would create crystal grids beside my bed and place specific symbols within the grids, depending upon the emotional issues I was facing. The energetic signatures of the symbols were carried in the crystalline vortex field and broadcast to me while I was in bed. This allowed me to clear my emotional complexes while I slept (see *Chapter 2*).

Waveform Symbols Used to Clear Mental/Emotional Tension

Between 1991 and 1993, I obtained a strong grounding in the application of the *Waveform Symbols*. I discovered that when I felt upset and out-of-sorts, I often could take the sharp edge off of my emotional state with the use of the symbols.

I also noticed that the *Waveform Symbols* frequently helped me clear the mental fog I had around some problem, allowing me to see the solution from a higher vantage point.

Using Waveform Symbols with Clients

Around 1993, I began using the *Waveform Symbols* in my spiritual consulting practice and discovered that my clients responded favorably to the symbol energies. The symbols helped my clients resolve their emotional traumas and upsets.

I developed a way to broadcast the essence of a symbol to a client by holding the card up (with the symbol facing him/her) and visualizing light beaming from my hand through the symbol card to him/her. As I do this, I hold the intention that the symbol's frequency fills the client's body and being (See *Chapter 3*). Many healings occurred using this approach.

Using Waveform Symbols in Spiritual Attunements

In 1993, I also began using the *Waveform Symbols* in spiritual attunements to assist individuals in aligning with the spiritual qualities expressed by the symbols.

Waveform spiritual attunements were incorporated in the musical album *Ascension Harmonics: Sacred Attunements Through Music*, in collaboration with the musician Richard Shulman. Richard experienced 16 Waveform initiations to which he spontaneously channeled music.

During the final mix of the album, I directed the specific *Waveform Symbol's* energy into the digital master recording, allowing the music and Waveform energies to merge as one.

My impression was that the music became the container and channel for the Waveform energies and that the Waveform frequencies, in turn, enhancing the listener's appreciation of the music (See *About the Author* section for information on the *Ascension Harmonics CDs.*)

Requests for a Waveform Symbol Card Deck

As I continued using my crudely drawn *Waveform Symbol* card deck with friends, relatives, and clients, many of them suggested that a professional card deck be made available to a wider audience.

At that time, I felt I did not have the artistic skill to create the polished symbol paintings I was envisioning. I approached several artists about collaborating on the Waveform deck, but for various reasons there was no interest. I realize in hindsight that the resistance occurred because I was not ready at that time for the intense emotional clearing I would experience in writing the descriptions of the symbols presented in this book.

Creating the Card Deck and Book

In January 1996, a friend, Stephen Lord, offered to assist me in the production of the *Waveform Symbol* card deck. He provided me some seed money which helped "kick start" my intention to create the card deck. After Stephen and I agreed on the format for the deck and its accompanying book, I reviewed the more than 200 *Waveform Symbols* I had accessed by 1996 and intuitively (through muscle testing) selected the 33 symbols to be used for the cards. I also muscle tested the numerical order for the symbols.

Both Stephen and I had expected the creation of the cards and this accompanying book to move quickly. We discovered, however, that the *Waveform Symbol* project had its own time schedule which did not adhere to our artificial deadlines.

Describing Each Waveform Symbol

Stephen and I spent many days, over a number of months, channeling the descriptions for each of the *Waveform Symbols*. To truthfully describe, as best as I could, the essence of each symbol, I found myself continually "attuning to" its energy.

Each symbol represents an ideal or perfected state of being. I felt the symbol's description needed to express those ideal qualities. This required invoking the symbol's frequencies, embodying them, then channeling the intuitive guidance received about the symbol.

I often experienced, however, that a childhood memory (a past choice or decision I had made and held in my subconscious) was in conflict with the ideal state represented by the symbol.

For example: Card #8, "I am loved. I love. I am love." If I had ever felt unloved, unworthy and unwanted, those memories would set up resistance to being in the state of love expressed in the essence of the symbol. The resistance always appeared to be cleared by the energy of the symbol, but only after it surfaced. That is, the vibration of the symbol transmuted the emotional charges that were in resistance.

However, the transmutation was not always instantaneous. The inner conflict took a little or sometimes a long time to clear. In healing lingo the clearing of inner resistance is called "processing"—and "process" I did.

On the average, it would take me two days of focusing on the pure essence of a symbol and to write a description of its qualities. If I had no subconscious conflict with the ideal expressed by the symbol, the writing flowed. When I did have resistance, it felt like I was pushing through mud to find the words to describe the symbol's qualities. I emotionally "processed" the frequencies of one specific symbol for over three weeks.

A Personal Purification

Although the clearing of my inner conflict was not necessarily a joyful experience, it initiated a significant healing within myself. As the weeks and months passed, and more symbol descriptions were completed, I found myself feeling lighter and much more at peace.

Friends of mine commented that my physical structure (e.g. my face) had started to regenerate and rejuvenate. I found myself moving deeper into the core of my Being and experiencing "no fear."

The Artist for the Waveform Symbol Card Deck

The exceptional artist of the *Waveform Symbol* paintings is Paul Bond. He took the hand drawn symbols and transformed them into works of art. Paul allowed himself to receive the energetic attunements of each of the *Waveform Symbols.*

In doing so, he was able to direct its energetic frequency via his air brush equipment into the symbol's shape/form when he painted it. Paul's love for his work played an important role in the power and quality of the *Waveform Symbol* card deck.

I worked with Paul to intuitively select the appropriate colors for the symbols and the colors for the background of each symbol. The colors selected were based on the chakras that the symbols affected.

Paul and I often recalibrated the shape of the symbol so that it carried the highest signature frequency. The process was fascinating. If we changed the size of a loop or a curve in a line in a particular symbol, that change would shift the Symbol's overall vibration.

Paul and I played with changing the shape of the symbol until its frequency felt correct. Sometimes we had to go through three or four iterations of the symbol's shape. When we arrived at the correct form, we often both knew that it was "the one."

Paul would then began painting the symbol.

Déjà Vu

The cards were first published in 2002, thirteen years after I first ventured into the Cave of Symbols/Ancients. As I stood by the printing press watching the freshly printed Waveform cards rolling off the press, I experienced a very strong déjà vu. I could feel the frequencies radiated off the symbol cards and I was once again standing in the Cave of Symbols. I felt I had returned home.

Ownership of the Waveform Symbols

I channeled these symbols but do not claim to be their creator. My Intuitive Self gifted me with the ability to access them, but I claim no ownership of them.

It is like someone gifting you with a library card, allowing you to access books from the library. However, your ability to access books is predicated on the library card. And your ability to access books does not mean you wrote the books.

Because of the time, effort, and money that went into creating the Waveform card deck, I do view the card deck as proprietary. However, I do not view the *Waveform Symbols* themselves as proprietary. I believe the symbols are universal and available to anyone. You are welcome to use your versions of the symbols. The universe grants you the permission to do so.

If you publish the Symbols or post them on your website, I respectfully ask that you mention where you obtained them (thanks).

The End of the Story?

The story continues on with you. The *Waveform Symbols* are

powerful healing tools which you can use daily in your life. And the more that you work with them, the more applications you will discover. Friends of mine, since acquiring their card deck, have religiously selected a card for that day. It is a practice that they say helps to guide them through their life.

The *Waveform Symbols* can support you as well. They can help you to meet life's challenges and vicissitudes. And they can also assist you in achieving your goals and manifesting your dreams. Such is their potential.

CHAPTER 1
Card for the Day and Self Balancing Card Spreads

Each *Waveform Symbol* has a specific frequency which can help clear and transmute trauma. Some of the symbols clear on the cellular and DNA level; others balance and align on an emotional and mental level. A card, or a series of symbol cards, can be selected to help you release emotional issues that arise, or to guide you to an area in your life that needs to be examined and healed.

The selection of the cards is always recommended to be done with the guidance of your Higher Self (*Source Essence*). This aspect of yourself knows all answers, sees future probabilities based upon present choices, and is aware of what is in your highest good. Choose to align with your Higher Self before selecting your cards to improve the accuracy of your symbol choices.

Card for the Day

Each day presents its own challenges, offers its unique individual lessons, and is bathed in its own astrological energies. Choosing a *"Card for the Day"* provides guidance as to what is up to be addressed, what issue would best be resolved, or what spiritual quality would serve you that day.

The *Waveform Symbols* differ from many card decks in that

the symbol cards can be used to help heal the issues pinpointed. Using intention, you can transfer the energy of the symbol to yourself to clear the emotional charge surrounding any issue.

Selecting and Using a "Card for the Day"

1. Shuffle the cards; spread them face down before you. **Note:** In some card decks, reversed or upside down cards carry a meaning. This is not the case with the Waveform cards.
2. Before selecting a "*Card for the Day*," it is suggested that you set the intention of connecting and aligning with your Higher Self. One powerful meditation technique is as follows:
    a. Close your eyes and relax.
    b. See a pool of light within your heart chakra that represents the essence of your Higher Self.
    c. Surrender and step into the light of your soul.
    d. Allow yourself to sink deep into this pool of light and merge with your soul essence.
3. Once you feel connected with the Source of your Being, ask, "*Beloved Higher Self, assist me in selecting the appropriate card for this day which carries the vibrational qualities which will support me in my growth and evolution.*"
4. With the cards lying face down (with the "*As above, so below*" side showing), select the card that appears to have the most energy. One approach is to scan the cards visually until one catches your eye. You can also hold your hand over the cards, slowly moving it over the spread until one card seems to jump out at you. You can also use muscle testing or a pendulum to select the card.
5. After selecting the "*Card for the Day*," reconnect with your soul essence and ask your Higher Self to show you the

relevance of the card. Here are some questions you can ask yourself:

a. Besides yourself, is there an individual or situation in your life that this card directly speaks to?

b. Is the symbol card pointing to a situation on your event horizon which may soon manifest? Do you want this situation to manifest? If not, is the symbol card suggesting a solution?

c. Is the card addressing a core emotion that needs to be healed?

Note: In this book, the description of each symbol has a subsection called "*Card for the Day.*" In the "*Card for the Day*" subsection the meaning of the symbol is discussed, as well as suggestions on how to use the symbol card in meditation.

6. The energetic essence of the symbol can be transferred to yourself through intention. This process can help you more fully embody the symbol's essence and come into alignment with its truth. The easiest way of doing this is as follows:

a. Hold the symbol card up to your heart chakra, with the actual symbol pointing toward your body.

b. Reconnect with your Higher Self and ask for the transfer of the highest frequencies of the symbol into all levels of your Being, bringing you into alignment with its essence.

c. Then, as you inhale, choose that the frequency of the symbol is infused in your body.

7. You may also want to consider placing the symbol card inside a crystal grid built beside your bed. In this manner, the vibration of the symbol can be broadcast to you, allowing you to unconsciously clear any emotional issues while you sleep. (See *Chapter 2: Waveform Card Grids.*)

Self-Balancing Card Spreads

Often, we find ourselves presented in life with emotional challenges and situations which can knock us off center. The *Waveform Symbol Cards* provide a tool to help us rise above our issues and transform our negative emotional states.

The foundational premise is that our Higher Self knows the next step we should take which is in our best interest. By asking your Higher Self for direction, you will receive the necessary guidance. If you take the time to align with your soul essence and ask for guidance, you will find yourself selecting the symbols that offer you a solution. Multiple symbol cards can be chosen to help you resolve any emotional issue that you are facing.

Suppose you have just lost a job, or a friend had a car accident, or failed a test. Or perhaps, you think you cannot do what you really want to do, or you must do something unpleasant. Whatever your issue, a self-balancing card spread can be conducted to clear the emotional charge and/or resistance.

Steps to Conducting a Self-Balancing Card Spread

1. You can select any number of cards when doing a self-balancing spread. The number of symbols selected is determined by your Higher Self and usually ranges from 1 to 7 cards, although any number is possible (up to 33 cards). The recommended procedure is to shuffle the cards and then spread them face down so you can see only the backside of the cards. The backside of the cards say, *"As above, so below."*

2. Choose to align with your Higher Self and then focus on the emotional issue for which you need relief or guidance. Ask your Higher Self to assist you in selecting the cards which will help you resolve or heal the problem.

3. Scan the cards visually or pass your hand over the cards. Select those symbol cards that appear to have an energetic charge or which seem to stand out when you visually focus upon them. You can also use muscle testing or a pendulum to select your cards.

4. After the cards are chosen, with the cards still face down, ask for guidance as to their correct order. Which card should I look at first? Which card should I look at second? And so on. When the cards have been rearranged in the appropriate order, it is time to study them face up.

   Note: There is often a surprising logic to the sequence of symbol cards selected, as if the affirmations for each card form a sentence or a paragraph. For an in-depth understanding of the message provided by your Higher Self, you may want to review the "*Insight*" section for each symbol selected.

5. The vibrational and energetic essence of each of the chosen symbols can now be transferred into your Being through intention. (**Note**: Since most self-balancing spreads have two or more symbol cards selected, you will discover there is a synergistic effect when a group of symbols are used. The total energetic impact from the group of symbol cards appears much stronger than from just one individual symbol card.)

   To transfer the symbol card energies through intention, follow these recommended steps:

   a. Again, choose to align with your Higher Self. Focus on your heart. Imagine a doorway into your heart chakra and pass through it. Once you are within your heart space, see a pool of light which represents your soul essence. Choose to surrender and step into the pool of light, sinking deep into the Source of your Being.

b. Once you feel fully connected with your soul essence, state: *"Beloved Higher Self, I ask that the highest frequencies and qualities of these symbols be transferred to me, clearing all emotional and mental charges. I now choose to move into balance and harmony. Furthermore, I choose to receive clarity as to my best course of action. So be it."*

c. Bring each card, in the sequence chosen, up to your heart chakra. Position the symbol so it is facing toward your body. As you inhale, visualize drawing the symbol's energy through your heart into your whole body. Imagine the color and vibration of the symbol filling you completely. When it feels that the energetic quality of the symbol is fully infused in your being, move on to the next symbol in the series.

You will often feel your emotional state shift as you conduct this process. In most cases you will feel calmer and more at peace when you complete the energetic transfer of all the symbol cards selected.

If the symbol card spread selected addresses a core issue for you, you may want to slowly soak in the vibrational essence of the symbols while you sleep. One powerful way of doing this is to create a crystal grid beside your bed, within which the selected symbol cards are placed. The grid will allow the vibrational essence of the symbols to be held in an energy field around you as you sleep. (See *Chapter 2, "Waveform Card Grids."*)

CHAPTER 2
Waveform Card Grids

Introduction

A crystal grid can be created by arranging six crystals in a Star of David pattern. The six crystals are positioned so that they define the vertices of two intersecting triangles. The arrangement of crystals in such a pattern generates an energy field that extends beyond the crystals. The energy field generated is a spinning vortex similar to a whirlpool.

When you place *Waveform Symbol Cards* inside the crystal grid, the grid's energy field begins to carry the vibrational frequencies of the symbols. In other words, the energy field generated by the grid carries the frequencies of the symbols placed within it. Thus, the energies of the *Waveform Symbols* can be broadcast at-a-distance through the grid's vortex.

If you place a *Waveform Symbol Grid* beside your bed, its vortex field will surround you while you sleep, allowing you to unconsciously absorb the symbol's frequencies. If you place a *Waveform Symbol* grid beneath a massage table, its vortex field will extend up through the table. The person lying on the table will, in this manner, be surrounded by the frequencies of the *Waveform Symbols*.

Using Waveform Grids While You Sleep

Approximately 1/3 of our lives is spent in sleep. During sleep we unconsciously focus on our unsolved problems and issues through our dreams. The time we spend in sleep each day is an auspicious time to use the *Waveform Symbols* to address and resolve emotional issues.

If you want to heal an emotional issue through the assistance of the *Waveform Symbols*, you can place the selected symbol cards inside a crystal grid by your bed. The symbol's frequencies will then be carried in the grid's energy field around you as you sleep. You can potentially resolve emotional issues during the dream state using this approach.

Waveform Grids in a Life Force Balancing Session

Reiki, acupressure, cranio-sacral and massage therapists can place Waveform crystal grids beneath the massage table so the symbol energies are present as they work with their clients. The clients can be asked to intuitively select the *Waveform Symbol Cards* to help them resolve their current issues. (Use the steps outlined in *Chapter 1*.)

The selected symbol cards can then be placed inside a Star of David crystal grid on the floor, just beneath the table. The energy field created by the crystal grid carries the *Waveform Symbol* frequencies up through the table and around the client during the session.

Firsthand experience using this approach has proven that symbol grids can readily assist clients in releasing their emotional and mental issues.

The Star of David Grid

I will be describing the creation of a Star of David grid shortly. The very shape of the Star of David, two inter–penetrating triangles, creates a vortex energy field. It should be noted that most symbols do not. The fact that the Star of David does generate a vortex makes it useful in broadcasting the *Waveform Symbol* frequencies.

The shape of the Star of David has been described as representing the balance of the masculine and feminine, sky and Earth energies. In numerology it is said to carry the value of "6," which resonates with the qualities of love, harmony and balance.

The vortex power of the Star of David grid is greatest when it is oriented along the magnetic North/South axis as shown in Figure #1.

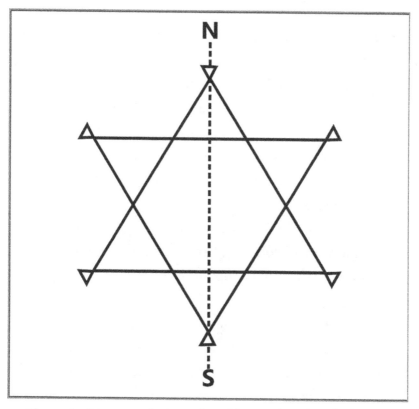

Figure #1: Diagram of a Star of David crystal grid with a North/ South magnetic axis running through it. Crystals are at each of the triangle vertices.

A compass, of course, will show you the magnetic North and South directions. It is recommended that the Star of David Grid be constructed so the apex of one of the triangles points directly to magnetic North, and the apex of the second triangle points due South.

Steps to Creating a Crystal Grid

1. Position six quartz crystals all at once on the floor so they serve as the vertices of the two interpenetrating triangles. Lay the crystals down in a clockwise fashion, directing the points of the crystals either all inward or all outward.

    Note: The kinds of crystals used to create the grids will affect the vibrational quality of the vortex field. Amethyst crystals, for example, will bring in the violet ray, citrine crystals, the gold-yellow ray. Clear quartz crystals are the best all-purpose crystals to use in constructing grids since they transmit White Light, and embody all color rays.

    However, you may want to experiment with different crystals. It is recommended that the color of the crystals selected match the primary, secondary, or tertiary color of the symbol(s) used within the grid.

    For example, if you have chosen a *Waveform Symbol* with a primary color of pink—a crystal grid built of pink rose quartz would help support the vibration of the symbol's frequency.

    In the description of each symbol is a list of additional crystals or metals which can be used in grid construction. These crystals or metals match the resonance of one of the colors of the symbol. The metals and crystals listed were selected based upon the chakras they activate.

2. Starting with the triad of crystals pointing to magnetic

North, direct the index finger of your dominant hand at the Northern-most pointing crystal.

3. Visualize brilliant white light shooting out of your fingers into the crystal, rather like a laser beam. When it feels as if the energy has "locked in" to the crystal, draw a line of Light in a clockwise fashion to the next crystal in the triangle.

4. Again, sense the energy as it "locks in" to the second crystal. Then draw a line of light to the third crystal in the triangle. When the energy is seated into the third crystal, draw a line of light back to the crystal you began with. To strengthen the energetic bonding, it is recommended that you loop through the three crystals three times, drawing lines of light as you do.

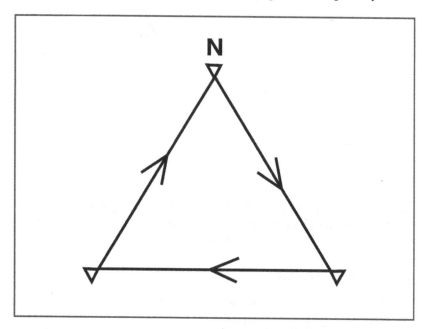

Figure #2. Diagram of an upward pointing triangle with a crystal at each of the three vertices of the triangle. The triangle points North.

Note: You have now defined a triangle with lines of light, where the three crystals are the vertices of the triangle. The crystals hold the lines of energy, or light, in place. Should the crystals be accidentally disrupted, the light lines will be broken and will have to be redrawn if you want the grid to be active.

It is suggested that you draw the lines of light in a clockwise manner, setting up a clockwise vortex which supports health and well-being.

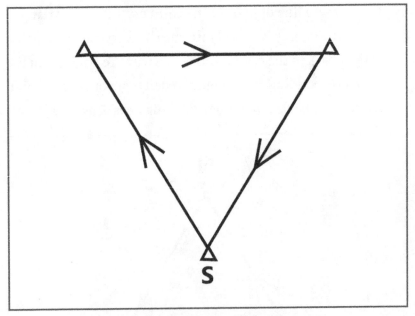

Figure #3. Diagram of a downward pointing triangle with a crystal at each of the three vertices of the triangle. The triangle points South.

5. Now, draw the lines of light in a clockwise manner between the three crystals of the second triangle—the triangle pointing south. To assure that the energy linkage is strong, link the three crystals, three separate times. After completing the last loop, choose to disconnect energetically from the grid.

6. The Star of David Grid is now complete. See Figure #4 on the facing page.

The Completed Star of David Grid

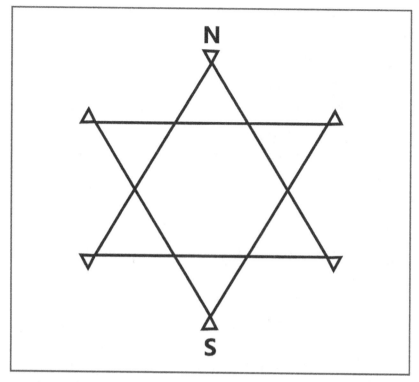

Figure #4. Diagram of both intersecting triangles of the Star of David grid. There ia a crystal at each of the six vertices of the two triangles. The grid is aligned along the North/South axis.

You are ready to add the *Waveform Symbol Cards* to the inside of the crystal grid. There can be any number of symbol cards added to the grid, but usually it is from 1 to 7. (See *Chapter 1 The Self-Balancing Spread* for details on the card selection process.)

6. Among the *Waveform Symbol Cards* you have selected for your grid, determine which card should go inside the grid first, which should go in second, and so on. (This step applies only if you are placing two or more symbol cards in the grid.)

7. Pick up the first symbol card selected for the grid and hold

it so the symbol faces upward, away from the floor. Begin moving the card above the grid in a large clockwise circle. Keep moving the card in a circle until you intuitively feel the best place to set it down within the grid. The right place will often feel more energetic—more alive. Set the card down inside the Star of David grid and rotate the card, face up, until the alignment feels good to you.

8. Continue this intuitive placement process for each of the symbol cards you plan to put inside the grid. That is:

    a. Pick up a card.

    b. Move it in a clockwise circle above the grid.

    c. Determine the location that feels best for placement of the card.

    d. Place the symbol card in that position, face up.

    e. Rotate the alignment of the card until it energetically feels correct.

After all the symbol cards are in place, their combined frequencies will be held within the crystal grid's energy field. Often a powerful synergistic effect is created when the frequencies of a number of symbols merge together. It is as if the card frequencies support each other exponentially, clearing and transmuting energy blocks more forcefully than if they were used individually.

Removal of the Grid

When you are ready to take the crystal grid down, it is recommended that you pick up the crystals in a clockwise fashion, starting with any of the crystals in the grid. Continue to circle around the grid clockwise, picking up each of the crystals.

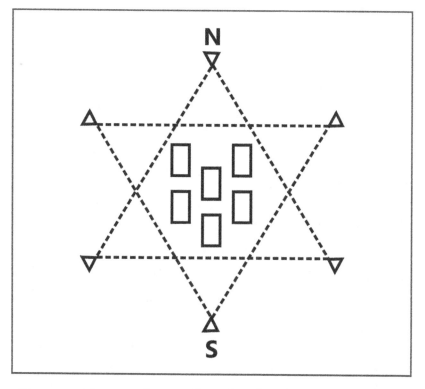

Figure #5. Diagram of a Star of David grid with Waveform Symbols within it.

Clearing Your Crystals

Be sure to clear your crystals after using them. They may have absorbed low-grade emotional frequencies while in the grid.

For example, when Waveform crystal grids are placed under a massage table and used in a balancing session, they often facilitate the rapid release of old emotional energies from the client.

The emotional frequencies of anger, fear, or grief (to name a few) can be released from the client's emotional body and enter the grid field to be picked up by the crystals.

Waveform grids set up by your bed can assist you in letting

go of old emotions while you sleep and these less-than-desirable frequencies can also become encoded into the crystals.

It is extremely important, therefore, to clear your grid crystals every time you use them so you don't bring the previously released emotional frequencies into your newly constructed Waveform grid. This is an extremely important point.

If you don't plan to clean your crystals, then please don't construct crystal grids!

A Simple Way to Cleanse Your Crystals

Clearing your crystals is surprisingly simple. Just place them on the deck of Waveform cards, where all the symbols in the deck are face up. Allow them to sit on top of the deck for a minimum of 15 minutes.

The *Waveform Symbols* will clear the crystals automatically. However, to enhance the clearing process, you can set an intention that the clearing occurs.

The *Waveform Symbols* are self-clearing and do not themselves require purification.

Note: The crystals can certainly sit longer than 15 minutes on the card deck. I have often let my crystals sit on a deck for hours or even days. Fifteen minutes is just the recommended minimum time period.

Besides being cleared of low-grade emotional frequencies, the crystals will also be encoded with the higher symbol frequencies of the deck.

CHAPTER 3
Energetic Balancing Using Colors and Waveform Symbols

The *Waveform Symbols* can be used as a powerful energetic balancing tool. The symbols assist in clearing the emotional charges and the mental issues that are suspected to be the basis of many physical ailments.

Used in this manner, the symbols serve as a disease preventative, helping to dissolve emotional and mental blockages before they manifest as physical disease symptoms.

The Transfer of the Symbol's Vibration through Intention

The phrase *"energy follows thought"* expresses the notion that what you focus upon becomes energized and amplified.

We are able to direct the flow of life force energy (also called chi, ki, prana, manna, or orgone) by directing our thoughts to an idea or object. Our intention becomes a lens which concentrates and directs the life force upon that which we are focused.

During a therapeutic session, the *Waveform Symbols* can be broadcast through intention and visualization to a friend or client to assist in his/her clearing and balancing. Three methods of transferring the frequencies of the symbols will now be discussed.

Method 1

Assuming your dominant hand is your right hand[1], hold the corner of the *Waveform Symbol* card in your left hand, with the symbol facing the person. The back of the card, which has the affirmation, *"As Above, So Below,"* will be facing you.

Now bring your right hand two to three inches behind the back of the card, with your palm facing the back of the card.

Visualize a beam of light directed out of your right palm, through the symbol card, and to the individual you are working with.

The beam of light can be any color you choose, although the primary, secondary, or tertiary colors of the specific *Waveform Symbol* are recommended.

As you visualize the beam of light passing through the symbol card to its recipient, silently affirm that the *"purest, clearest and highest frequencies of the symbol be transferred."*

Choose that the vibrations of the symbol are carried within the colored beam and infused into the person.

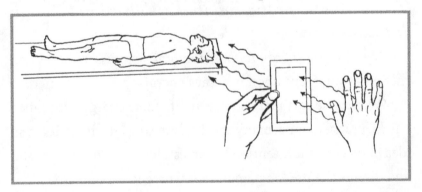

Figure #6. Hold a Waveform card in your left hand and direct energy out the right hand (through the card) to the client.

---

1 **Note***: If your dominant hand is left, hold the symbol card in your right hand and project the light beam out of your left hand through the symbol card.*

Method 2

Again, assuming your dominant hand is the right hand, hold the *Waveform Card* in the palm of your right hand. The back of the card with the affirmation, *"As Above, So Below,"* is hidden from view, as it lies in your palm. The symbol and its affirmation can be seen cupped in your palm.

Hold your right hand and arm pointed to the recipient. Simultaneously hold your left hand, palm up. Visualize light entering both your left palm and the crown of your head. Feel the light flowing through your body and exiting your right hand.

Imagine a beam of light projected out of your right hand, passing through the symbol card to the individual. The light beam can be different colors based upon the chakras you wish to activate (more on this later).

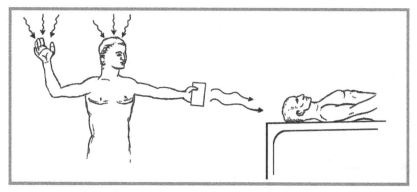

Figure #7. Holding a card in your right hand and your left hand held up in the air, draw energy in through your crown and left hand and direct the energy out your right hand (through the card) to the client.

Silently choose, as you direct the light to its recipient, that the *"purest, clearest, and highest frequencies of the symbol be transferred."* Visualize and feel the symbol's frequency being carried on the ray of light and infused into the individual.

Method 3

The *Waveform Symbol Cards* can also be placed directly on a friend or client while they are lying down. The symbols will have the greatest influence if they are placed on the major chakras of the body (to be discussed shortly).

When placing the cards on the body, lay them so the symbol faces the skin and the back of the card with the affirmation, "As Above, So Below," faces upward. It is recommended that the symbol's primary or secondary colors match the color that activates the chakra upon which it is placed.

For example, the colors that help activate the heart chakra are green, turquoise, pink or gold. If you use any of the *Waveform Symbols* which have the colors of green, turquoise, pink, or gold, then those symbols would help open and clear the heart chakra.

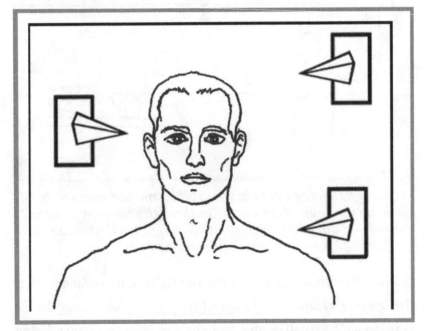

Figure #8. Crystals lying on symbol cards which point to the crown, brow and throat chakras of someone lying face up on a massage table.

(**Note**: The colors associated with each chakra will be described later in this chapter.)

After you have intuitively selected the Waveform *Symbol Cards* and are about to lay them over the chakra centers of the recipient, connect your Higher Self to the Higher Self of the individual and silently request that "*the purest, clearest, and highest frequencies of the symbol be used by the individual for his/her highest good.*"

Suggestion: Since it is difficult to lay the cards on the crown, brow, or throat chakras, the symbol cards can be laid on the massage table close to the head of the individual when working with these upper chakras. Clear quartz crystals can be placed on the symbols and directed toward the chakras for which they are intended. (See Figure #8 on the facing page.)

Using the Waveform Symbols in a Balancing Session

Ask your Divine Self these questions when you are about to conduct a Life Force Balancing session such as Reiki, acupressure, polarity, or similar modality:

1. Which *Waveform Symbols* would best be placed within crystal grids beneath the massage table (See *Chapter 2*)?
2. Which symbols would be most effective placed on the chakras?
3. Which symbols would be most appropriate to broadcast with the currents of light (*Methods #1* or *#2*) at the beginning of the session?

If you place the 33 *Waveform Symbols* face up on a table near you as you work, you can easily view the symbols as the session progresses. Then as emotional layers come up to be cleared during the session, you can access the appropriate symbols and broadcast them to the recipient as outlined in *Method #1* and *Method #2.*

The Major Chakras and Their Associated Colors

Our body's energy centers, known as chakras, have been described exceptionally well in Barbara Ann Brennan's two books, *Hands of Light—a Guide to Healing Through the Human Energy Field,* and *Light Emerging—The Journey of Personal Healing.* The reader is referred to these books for descriptive illustrations and prose on the shape and function of the chakras.

The term *"chakra"* is a Sanskrit word meaning *"spinning wheel,"* for this is how the chakras appeared to the clairvoyants of ancient India. They are vortex energy centers where the life force (chi, ki, prana, manna) is pumped into and out of the body. There are major and minor chakras feeding the life force energy to all the organs, glands, muscles and tissues in the body.

The more expansive and faster spinning the vortex chakra center, the more life force energy is pumped by the chakra and generally the healthier the organs and tissues associated with that chakra. However, emotional and mental issues can become stuck in a chakra causing its spin to slow down and its field of influence to contract.

When this happens, the amount of life force available to the organs and tissues around the chakra drops. With the decrease in vitality, what we normally describe as disease (dis-ease or lack of ease) can set in (e.g., loss of tissue structure, viral or bacterial infection).

A table of the seven major chakras, their location, and some of the organs and glands associated with each chakra is shown

CHAKRAS AND GLANDS
SEVEN MAJOR CHAKRAS AND ASSOCIATED GLANDS

CHAKRA	LOCATION	ASSOCIATED GLAND
Crown	Top of the head	Pineal
Brow	Forehead	Pituitary, brain, eyes
Throat	Throat	Thyroid, parathyroid (metabolism)
Heart	Center of chest	Heart, thymus, lungs
Solar Plexus	Below sternum	Pancreas, liver, gall bladder, spleen, stomach, ileocecal valve, colon, duodenum, appendix
Sexual (sacral)	Over pubic bone	ovaries/uterus, testes/prostrate, bladder, colon
Root (base)	Base of tail bone	Adrenals, kidneys, coccyx, rectum

above.[2]

The lungs, for example, are associated with the heart chakra. If someone is suffering a lung ailment, such as asthma, this strongly suggests that the heart chakra is not operating at full capacity, circulating the necessary life force through the lungs. Of course, there could be many other complications involved. However, a diminished heart chakra would mean reduced vitality in both the lungs and thymus, thereby weakening the body's ability to open the lungs and regenerate the lung tissues.

Issues of the heart, such as a broken romance, not feeling loved, or not loving oneself (self-judgment), can slow down the

---

2 **Note:** *Many sources describing the higher chakras agree on the correlated glands, organs, and locations. However, there are varied opinions concerning the lower chakras. The following chart includes location of the glands and organs for the lower (root, sexual, solar plexus) chakras based upon personal experience working with the energy bodies of my clients.*

spin rate of the heart chakra (vortex), in turn affecting the vitality of the physical heart, thymus (master gland of the immune system), and the lungs.

The *Waveform Symbols* can assist in addressing the emotional issues being held in the chakras, thereby potentially clearing those blockages from the chakras and increasing the vitality, regeneration, and rejuvenation of the associated organs.

The *Waveform Symbols* do not heal or cure disease; rather, they work vibrationally to bring harmony to our emotional and mental issues and can, therefore, help resolve the inner conflict which first sets the stage for the manifestation of disease.

Chakra Colors

Specific colors will help activate, stimulate and open the seven major chakras. These colors can be invoked, visualized, and broadcast as a beam of light, along with the frequency of the *Waveform Symbol*, to a friend or client. The visualized beam of light (described in *Methods #1* and *#2*) acts as a carrier wave for the symbol's vibration to synergistically enhance the positive effect of the *Waveform Symbol*.

The colors listed in the chart below help to vitalize and acti-

COLORS RELATED TO CHAKRAS		
CHAKRA	SPECTRUM	NON-SPECTRUM
crown chakra	violet	(purple, gold)
brow chakra	indigo	(cobalt blue)
throat chakra	blue	(turquoise)
heart chakra	green	(turquoise, pink, gold)
solar plexus chakra	yellow	(lemon)
sexual chakra	orange	(reddish-orange)
root chakra	red	(pink)

vate the seven major chakras:

As a general rule, the primary color (the actual color of the symbol, not its background color) for each *Waveform Card* indicates the chakra it influences the most. For example, if a specific *Waveform Symbol* has the greatest effect on the solar plexus chakra, then its primary color will be yellow or lemon. If a *Waveform Symbol* directly influences the throat chakra, its primary color will be blue, and so on.

The secondary and tertiary colors of the symbol reflect the other chakras that are also positively influenced by that specific symbol. For example, *Waveform Symbol Card #1* (*"I Release All Doubt And Walk In Faith."*) has red as its primary color, yellow its secondary color, and reddish orange as its tertiary color.

Thus, this symbol positively affects the root chakra (red), the solar plexus chakra (yellow), and the sexual chakra (reddish orange). This particular symbol helps to activate and open the three lower chakras, promoting "grounding" and the clearing of the fear vibration into the Earth.

Methods #1 and *#2* describe the visualization and broadcasting of a symbol's frequency on a beam of light. Although any of an infinite number of colors could be broadcast along with the symbol's frequency, it is recommended that the colored ray of light visualized match either the primary, secondary, or tertiary color for the symbol.

For example, *Symbol Card Number 1*, just mentioned, could effectively be broadcast on a beam of red, yellow, or reddish orange light.

The description of each symbol includes a subsection called *"Color and Symbol Balancing."* Suggestions are provided in this subsection as to the colors to visualize and broadcast with the symbol when using *Methods #1* and *#2* in a session. As a quali-fying statement, know that none of these suggested colors are "carved in stone," and if you are guided to use an entirely differ-ent colored ray, then by all means do so.

Visualization of Colors

The metaphysical perspective sees an ocean of etheric "life force" that interpenetrates our physical world. Everything that has mass, substance, or some kind of form has a reflected image of itself in the etheric dimension (and visa versa). Also, anything vibrating on the physical plane sets up similar harmonic vibra-tions on the etheric plane.

Thus, the electromagnetic frequencies of light you define as color have those same color frequencies set in motion in the etheric energy field. If, for example, you broadcast blue light with a light projector, you are simultaneously transmitting the frequency of blue on the etheric level.

The etheric energy field can also be directed and shaped through consciousness as exemplified by the miracles of the Masters. When you set the intention of visualizing a colored beam of light broadcast to a person, that conscious intention focuses and shapes the etheric field so the individual receives an etheric representation of that colored ray.

Over time, as you becomes practiced and adept in visualiz-ing different colored rays of light, the impact of the visualized color will become more pronounced. The individuals receiving the etheric colors will often be able to see the projected color in their mind's eye and to speak about the changes they are expe-riencing in their body.

They respond as if the actual colored light had been physically projected upon their skin. Thus, visualizing the projection of colored rays to a friend or client (as in *Methods #1* and *#2*) has an effect similar to actually projecting those colors with a light projector.

The Effects of Different Colors

Perhaps the most extensive researcher in color therapy in recent history was Dinshah P. Ghadiali (1873-1966). He spent close to 60 years using colors to assist in his clients' healing. His research and approach are discussed in *Let There Be Light* and in the *Spectro-Chrome-Metry Encyclopaedia, Vols. 1-3.*

The following descriptions of the effects of various colors are largely drawn from his findings. Although Dinshah used light projectors to broadcast his color treatments, his discoveries on the influence of color are also applicable to colors projected through visualization and intention.

Spectrum Colors

VIOLET (ACTIVATES AND OPENS THE CROWN CHAKRA)

- assists in the clearing and purification of virus and bacterial infections
- helps to rebalance the nervous/electrical system of the body through maintenance of the potassium/sodium equilibrium
- stimulates the spleen/leukocyte production
- has a calming effect and can enhance meditative states
- helps to open and expand the life force energy flow throughout the subtle energy bodies (etheric, emotional, mental, and spiritual)
- has a cleansing and antiseptic quality on the physical, etheric, and other energy levels

INDIGO (ACTIVATES AND OPENS THE BROW CHAKRA)
- has a calming and relaxing effect on the emotional body
- helps to balance the hemispheres of the brain and assists in bringing harmony and balance between the left and right sides of the body
- strengthens the lymphatic and immune systems of the body, e.g. helps to increase phagocyte production in the spleen
- helps in the detoxification of the blood
- has a cooling and astringent effect
- assists the body in regulating and utilizing minerals
- helps in the treatment of face and head conditions (eyes, ears, sinuses, etc.)
- can help activate and awaken spiritual intuitive insight

BLUE (ACTIVATES AND OPENS THE THROAT CHAKRA)
- has a cooling, soothing, and relaxing effect on the body, reducing nervous excitement
- helps in treating conditions of the throat
- activates the thyroid gland
- has a tonic effect on the blood
- helps to relieve inflammatory diseases
- assists in the detoxification of the body
- strengthens the respiratory system
- increases vitality and metabolism
- helps the body rebuild, promotes growth
- has anti-carcinogenic qualities

GREEN (ACTIVATES AND OPENS THE HEART CHAKRA)
- strengthens the action of the thymus, enhancing immunity

- balances and harmonizes the whole physical body
- helps to lower blood pressure and balance the physical heart
- is an emotional stabilizer, calming and soothing
- assists in the relief of inflamed conditions
- helps in the detoxification of organs
- re-vitalizes conditions of exhaustion
- has antiseptic and purifying qualities

YELLOW (ACTIVATES AND OPENS THE SOLAR PLEXUS CHAKRA)
- stimulates and cleanses the liver, intestines and gastrointestinal tract
- can help relieve constipation
- activates the lymphatic system and purifies the blood
- assists in clearing digestive and stomach problems
- helps to enhance mental clarity and stimulates one's mental capacity
- indirectly strengthens nerves and the brain
- helps to awaken optimism, confidence, and joy in someone who feels despondent

ORANGE (ACTIVATES AND OPENS THE SEXUAL CHAKRA)
- enhances the functions of the spleen and pancreas
- helps in the detoxification of the colon
- helps relieve constipation
- assists in food assimilation and helps to balance the eliminative system
- helps to energize and revitalize the physical body
- can help in treating conditions of the sexual organs
- has an anti-spasmodic effect and can be used to calm

muscle spasms or cramps
- strengthens the etheric body

RED (ACTIVATES AND OPENS THE ROOT CHAKRA)
- stimulates the circulation of the blood and helps support the creation of hemoglobin
- helps to warm the body through blood circulation
- awakens the physical life force and strengthens one's will
- energizes the physical body, the liver, and muscular system
- helps to clear congestion and mucous

Non-Spectrum Colors

GOLD (ACTIVATES AND OPENS THE HEART, CROWN AND HIGHER CHAKRAS—ABOVE THE HEAD)
- strengthens the thymus gland and positively influences the immune system and its ability to resist disease
- helps to balance and harmonize the physical heart
- esoterically represents the Christ Ray; brings harmony and equilibrium to the spiritual and physical bodies
- opens the crown and higher chakras, supporting an emotional sense of unity and well-being

PURPLE (ACTIVATES AND OPENS THE CROWN CHAKRA AND THE CHAKRAS ABOVE THE CROWN)
- has a strong purification quality in the mental and emotional bodies
- enhances the functions of the veins
- acts like a vasodilator, lowering blood pressure
- induces relaxation
- tends to lower body temperature (antipyretic)

TURQUOISE (ACTIVATES AND OPENS THE HEART AND THROAT CHAKRAS)

- carries the purifying and balancing qualities of the color green, and the cooling and antiseptic qualities of the color blue
- enhances the growth of new skin which has been burned; acts as a skin tonic
- can help cool and calm any inflammation
- helps to bring harmony and balance to the body on all levels
- helps to calm overactive mental functions, e.g., mental burnout
- strengthens the respiratory system and helps to diminish respiratory problems such as chest colds, bronchitis and asthma

PINK (ACTIVATES AND OPENS THE HEART AND ROOT CHAKRAS)

- helps to bring comfort to the emotional body when feelings of unworthiness, anger, or heartbreak arise
- strengthens the feelings of love and compassion for oneself and others
- opens the heart and activates the thymus gland, thereby enhancing the immune system
- stimulates the rejuvenation of new tissues and skin

SILVER (ACTIVATES AND OPENS THE LOWER CHAKRAS)

- esoterically represents the Divine Mother and Divine Feminine
- helps to ground, center and align you with the Earth's magnetic energy

- balances the feminine energies, e.g. the left side of the body, the yin meridians
- supports one's receptive, intuitive nature

The Energy Bodies and Associated Colors

The different energetic levels of a person are called energy bodies. They are superimposed over each other and vibrate at different frequencies. However, they are also interdependent because there is cross-communication between one energy body and the next. They could be thought of as different vibrational aspects of Self.

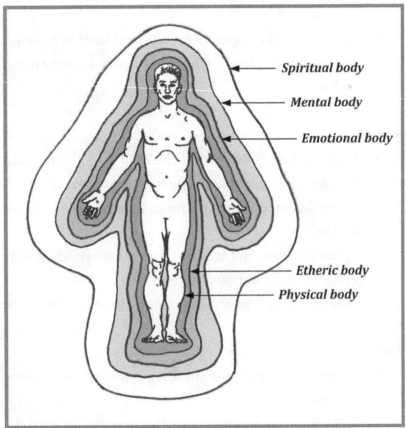

Figure #9. Drawing of the different energy bodies.

A general description of these energy bodies follows:

The Physical Body

This is the energy body you are most acquainted with. It is at the densest vibrational level—matter expressed in form as DNA, cells, tissues, organs, and glands.

The Etheric Body

This is the energetic level that holds the blueprint for our physical form. Templates for all structural, cellular and tissue components are encoded and held within the etheric body. Clairvoyants see the boundary layer of the etheric body approximately one to three inches above the skin.

The Emotional Body

This is the vibrational domain where our emotions, emotional complexes and charges are held. Here you carry at one time or another love, bliss, anger, guilt, fear, rage, and envy as energetic frequencies. The emotional body is at a higher vibrational frequency than the etheric and physical bodies. The boundary layer of the emotional body usually extends approximately 7 inches to five feet beyond the skin.

The Mental Body

The frequency of the mental body is a higher vibration than the emotional, etheric or physical bodies. This is the energy field holding our thoughts, thought forms, and mental conflict ("Yes, I am worthy" versus "No, I am not worthy"). The mental body's boundary layer usually extends approximately 15 inches to eight feet from the skin.

The Spiritual Body

This energy body encompasses the most expansive levels of consciousness and awareness, e.g., the knowing of the soul, the Divine Self or God-self. Some authors view the spiritual body as having additional layers such as the Monadic, Buddhic and Angelic levels, reflecting refinement in qualities of unity and God-awareness. The spiritual body's vibration is higher than that of the mental, emotional, etheric or physical bodies. Its boundary layer usually extends approximately 50 inches to about twelve feet beyond the skin. (It can extend for miles for enlightened beings.)

The vibrational healing paradigm suggests that all matter begins its formation at higher, more rarefied energy levels and then densifies into physical form.

If a diseased state exists on the physical level, there exists a diseased blueprint on a higher vibratory energy level. The clearing of the diseased blueprint allows the physical body to come back into balance and to heal itself (meaning "to make whole").

Visualized and projected colors and *Waveform Symbols* work vibrationally on the higher energy bodies such as the mental, emotional and etheric, allowing for the clearing of conflicted and blocked energy patterns which can manifest as disease.

Clearing of random, chaotic, and diseased energy patterns in the higher energy bodies (e.g. mental conflict held in the mental body) will cascade down creating a clearing at the lowest vibrational level—the physical body.

Each energy body has a set of colors with which it resonates most strongly, and which impacts it most significantly. The colors energizing our energy bodies are listed on the facing page.

COLOR ENERGETICS

ENERGY BODIES	VITALIZED BY THE COLORS
The Spiritual Body	gold, purple, violet, indigo, blue
The Mental Body	yellow, lemon, gold, blue, and turquoise
The Emotional Body	pink, orange, red, gold, and green
The Physical Body	green, turquoise

The Sacred Core Meditation Visualization

Some of the symbols have the "Sacred Core" visualization recommended in either the "*Meditation*" or "*Color And Symbol Balancing*" sections. The visualization is simple but very powerful. It involves seeing a pillar of light (e.g., white, gold, electric blue) running through the central axis of your body, including the spine. The top of the pillar of light extends up to the Great Central Sun, visualized at the center of the Universe, symbolically representing the Divine Father aspect.

The bottom of the light pillar extends down to the core of the Earth, which symbolically represents the Divine Mother aspect. Since the pillar of Light is unifying the Divine Father and Mother aspects within you, you represent the Divine Child.

The Sacred Core Visualization

This visualization helps to harmoniously integrate the seven major chakras. The visualization also assists in the balance and alignment of the physical, etheric, emotional, mental and spiritual bodies.

Furthermore, it helps to open the flow of life force energy through the entire body on all levels. The more often you practice the Sacred Core Meditation, the more effective it will become for you.

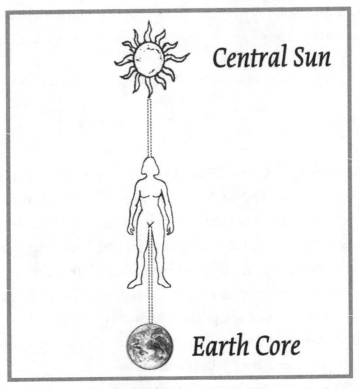

Figure #10. A column of light passing vertically through the body. One end of the light column connects to Central Sun, the other end to Earth Core.

Bibliography for Chapter 3

Amber, Reuben. *Color Therapy.* Aurora Press, Santa Fe, New
Mexico, 1983

Andrews, Ted. *The Healer's Manual: A Beginner's Guide to Vibrational Therapies.* Llewellyn Publications, St. Paul, Minnesota,
1993

Clark, Linda. Yvonne Martine. *Health, Youth and Beauty Through
Color Breathing.* Celestial Arts Berkeley, California, 1976

Dinshah, Darius. *Let There Be Light.* Dinshah Health Institute,
Malaga, New Jersey, 1985

Ghadiali, Dinshah P., *Spectro-Chrome-Metry Encyclopaedia, Vols.
1-3.* Spectro-Chrome Institute, New Jersey, 1939

Klotsche, Charles. *Color Medicine, The Secrets of Color/Vibrational
Healing.* Light Technology Publishing, Sedona, Arizona, 1995

Liberman, Jacob. *Light, Medicine of the Future.* Bear and Company, Santa Fe, New Mexico, 1991

CHAPTER 4
The Symbol Card Descriptions

A common format is followed for each of the *Waveform Symbol* descriptions:

Affirmation

A statement is provided that expresses the symbol's energy.

Insight

An expanded description of the symbol is discussed.

Card for the Day

After selecting a *"Card for the Day"* (See *Chapter 1*), you will find guidance in this subsection as to how the symbol's meaning might apply to your present circumstances.

Meditation

A visualization is provided in this subsection guiding you in transferring the symbol's vibration into your body/being for the purposes of clearing, purification and spiritual enhancement.

Color and Symbol Balancing

Different colored rays of light can be projected along with the symbol's frequency in an energy balancing session. This subsection outlines recommended colors and visualization approaches to use in such a session. The information presented in *Chapter 3, Energetic Balancing Using Colors and Waveform Symbols*, is a good introduction to this kind of energy balancing work.

Correspondences

Colors

The primary, secondary and tertiary colors of the symbol are listed. The specific colors of each symbol activate and balance certain chakras and energy bodies. (An in-depth description of the effects of various colors is provided in *Chapter 3*.)

Metals/Crystals Used in Grids

Certain crystals and metals have frequencies that harmonically support and amplify the symbol's colors and vibration. These crystals/metals are listed in this subsection for potential use in crystal grids. See *Chapter 2 ,Waveform Card Grids*, for a description on how to create crystal grids for broadcasting symbol frequencies.

Chakras Cleared and Aligned

The dominant chakras affected by the symbol are listed in this subsection. The chakras are listed in the order of the ones most strongly affected to those least affected. See *Chapter 3, Energetic Balancing Using Colors and Waveform Symbols*, for a description of the seven major chakras and their location on the body.

Meridians Cleared and Aligned

The primary meridians activated by the symbol are listed in this subsection. This information is provided for those readers acquainted with the meridian system. Further description of the twelve meridians (The "channels" through which the life force energy flows within the body) is beyond the scope of this book. For more details, review any acupuncture or acupressure book.

Primary Elements Represented by the Symbol

The elements represented by the symbol's essence are provided for those readers acquainted with the element theory and its use in the description of the action and effect of herbs, food and polarity circuits in the body. Generally, the qualities of the five elements are:

QUALITIES OF THE FIVE ELEMENTS	
ELEMENTS	QUALITIES
Ether	pre-matter, non-physical, high frequency
Air	vaporous, rapid change, mental
Fire	kinetic, hot, expanding outward, emotional-extrovert
Water	liquid, free flowing, cool, condensing inward, emotional-introvert
Earth	contracting, physical, solid, low frequency

A symbol may represent a number of elements simultaneously. If this is the case, the elements will be listed left to right, from the most dominant to the least dominant.

For example, *Card #7, I Look Within for Divine Wisdom* represents the energies of three primary elements: *Air/Fire/Water*, where *Air* is the most dominant element and *Water* is the least dominant, or least influential, element.

CARD #1

I Release All Doubt. I Walk in Trust and Faith.

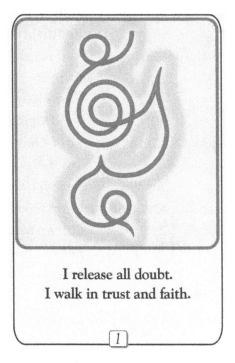

I release all doubt.
I walk in trust and faith.

1

AFFIRMATION:

"I know I am completely supported by the universe and this truth is fully grounded into my being."

Insight:

There are many levels to this symbol. First is trusting yourself and your connection to all things and all possibilities. It involves an awareness of other kingdoms (elemental, mineral, plant, animal, celestial), and your ties to them. Second is achieving a strong sense of your heart's desire and a knowing that it will manifest. Third involves a personal choice to ground your Self, as well as your desire, into physical form and the Earth plane.

CORRESPONDENCES

PRIMARY COLOR	Red
SECONDARY COLOR	Yellow
TERTIARY COLOR	Reddish-Orange
METALS\CRYSTALS USED IN GRIDS:	Red Jasper
	Garnet
	Carnelian
	Gold Yellow Citrine
CHAKRAS CLEARED AND ALIGNED:	Root Chakra
	Solar Plexus Chakra
	Sexual Chakra
MERIDIANS CLEARED AND ALIGNED:	Stomach Meridian
	Spleen Meridian
	Pericardium Meridian
	Liver Meridian
PRIMARY ELEMENTS REPRESENTED BY THE SYMBOL:	Earth/Water/Fire

Fourth is a willingness to let go of all thoughts and beliefs about limitation. For example, something cannot happen or cannot be accomplished.

The universe is a wondrous place, continually supporting you, giving you exactly what you want. It is rather like a "Yes Man" or a "Yes Woman" agreeing with your choices and assisting you in their manifestation. If you choose success, the universe says "yes" and you receive success. If you fear failure, the universe also says "yes," and you manifest failure. The life you are experiencing is an outward reflection of your beliefs and choices.

Doubt carries a hidden assumption that "it will not happen" or "it will not manifest." Doubt is yet another form of separation, a belief that you are disconnected from what you desire. It could be considered insidious, for the universe will support your belief in separation and the belief that you can't get what you want, just as it would support beliefs of wholeness and that you can have what you desire. You will be supported according to your beliefs.

Only by walking in faith and trust can you fully manifest your Divine Power. This requires commitment. It involves moving into alignment with the universe and re-directing your focus to your soul's love and away from all fear. In making a choice to manifest your heart's desire, you immerse yourself in the knowing that it has already manifested on an energetic level and merely needs to solidify into form. In doing so, you override any previous decision to disown your power.

The belief in miracles, the faith that every question will be answered and all desires fulfilled, is perhaps the most powerful and courageous level of awareness that can be maintained. It runs counter to the world's view of isolation from Source, of limitation, powerlessness, and lack. It aligns with the knowing that you are divine. With such faith, the magic of the magi and the wonder of the heavens can unfold on a daily basis.

Faith embodies more than just belief. In faith comes a knowing at the gut level (solar plexus chakra) and at the survival level (root or base chakra) that you are supported. With faith, nothing can ultimately hinder the manifestation of your desire. Faith is a feeling within your physical being that you are worthy of all your desires moving to completion. To walk in faith is to walk in your power and magic as a co-creator of your life.

Card for the Day:

If you selected this card, you may be feeling as if you are being tested and challenged. Take a deep breath and relax. Even the worst storm passes, leaving the air clean, clear and bright. To be fearless merely means to be without fear. Fear and doubt do not serve us and usually keep us from achieving what we desire.

Choose to cast all doubt aside and walk in trust and faith. Allow the emotions of fear or doubt to flow out from your feet into the Earth with each step you take. Align with the truth that you are supported by the universe. Each day is ripe with new potentialities and possibilities, and change is always a certainty.

Meditation:

Find a secluded spot. Study the symbol's shape and color. Hold the symbol card up to your heart (the symbol facing your body) and ask, "*Beloved Divine Self, I choose now to transmute all fear and doubt. I ask that the clearest and highest frequencies of this symbol fill me and allow me to walk in the faith and certainty that I am supported by the Source of my Being. So be it. And so it is!*"

Feel the colors and essence of the symbol flow into your heart and then through your entire body. Feel your strong bond with the Earth. Imagine yourself walking and letting go of all doubt and fear through your feet into the Earth. As these old emotional energies flow out, feel the hope and excitement that comes when your wish is fulfilled. Allow yourself the freedom to immerse yourself in the joy and wonderment of the full manifestation of your heart's desire.

Color and Symbol Balancing:

The three colors associated with this symbol assist in opening the lower three chakras and grounding your vision into physical reality.

Red is the primary color, which activates the base chakra, the energy center for grounding one into the physical plane. Red helps stimulate the biological life force and physical vitality held in the root chakra. It is difficult to manifest your goals in the world when the first chakra is closed down.

Yellow, the secondary color, helps you to expand and clear the solar plexus chakra, where issues of fear and doubt are often stored.

Reddish-Orange, the tertiary color of the symbol, helps you transmute and to clear separation from others through the expansion of the sexual chakra.

When using the symbol to balance another individual, it is recommended that the symbol's vibration be transmitted first on the Red Ray, then Yellow and finally the Reddish-Orange Ray. When transmitting with the Red Ray, see an aura of red light around the base chakra and visualize the chakra expanding like a red rose. Set the intention, as you do this, that the recipient feels comfortable being on the Earth and in his or her body.

Follow with a ray of bright yellow light. See it filling and infusing the solar plexus. Visualize the yellow light burning away any dark blockages in the solar plexus chakra. Hold the intention as you project the Yellow Ray that all "doubt" is transmuted to "faith."

When the solar plexus feels clear, broadcast the symbol's frequency on a current of reddish-orange light. Visualize the whole body infused with and radiating reddish-orange light. Choose that the infinite joyful energy of the universe energize and re-vitalize the individual.

CARD #2

I Accept Myself as Divine

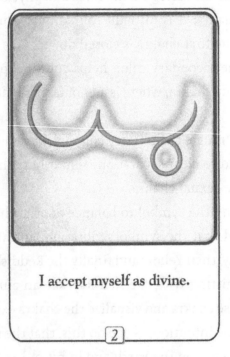

I accept myself as divine.

2

AFFIRMATION:

"I acknowledge and embody my divinity."

Insight

You are divine. Your divinity is an inherent part of your being, regardless of your beliefs about yourself. At one time millions of people believed the world was flat. However this misconception did not alter the truth. Likewise, believing you are separate from Source does not make it so. If you are experiencing limiting emotions like fear, anger, bitterness, or guilt, you are coming from the belief that you are alone and isolated. As real as these emotions appear, they nevertheless stem from a false assumption that you

CORRESPONDENCES

PRIMARY COLOR	Sky Blue
SECONDARY COLOR	Gold
TERTIARY COLOR	Purple
METALS\CRYSTALS USED IN GRIDS:	Aquamarine
	Blue Tourmaline
	Celestite
	Chrysocolla
	Gem Silica
CHAKRAS CLEARED AND ALIGNED:	Brow Chakra
	Crown Chakra
	Throat Chakra
MERIDIANS CLEARED AND ALIGNED:	Urinary/Bladder Meridian
PRIMARY ELEMENTS REPRESENTED BY THE SYMBOL:	Air/Water

are NOT divine and united with All-That-Is.

Accepting your divinity is necessary to fully manifesting your Divine Nature. Ultimately, you need to forgive yourself for choosing to feel separate from Source. The choice to feel separate usually begins in childhood, often in the womb, as a reaction to emotional pain expressed by your parents. Feeling dishonored, abandoned or unloved as a child leads to the belief that you are separate from your inner Divine Nature.

Your relationship with your parents is very often transferred to your relationship with God. If you feel your physical father did not support you, an unconscious belief that your Divine Father also does not support you is created. If you believe your physical mother did not honor you, there will be difficulty honoring yourself and grounding your energy into Mother Earth.

Being powerful is often portrayed in Western culture through control or manipulation of others. However, in the highest sense, "coming into your power" involves accepting your own divinity and allowing your divine capabilities to manifest in your life. One of the most powerful states of awareness is to accept the Divine Source of your Being as your True Nature and to choose to fully express your Divine Essence in your life.

Accepting yourself as divine inherently involves seeing others as divine and equal as well. Acknowledging your divinity is recognizing your unity with everyone in your life. It is a movement toward *At-One-Ment* and away from isolation. You attempt to control and regulate your life when you feel out of control, in fear, and "less than". When you can accept your divinity and unity with the Universal Flow, the need for control drops away, as does the need for pretense and glamour. You cannot be any greater, better, or more beautiful than you already are: a Divine Expression of the Universe.

Being fully centered in your divinity is also predicated on loving yourself and knowing at the deepest levels that you are "Okay." As you embody your sense of unity with the Source of your Being, there comes a knowing that you are worthy of the abundance of the universe, of friends, of love and support. As you tap into and accept your Divine and Infinite Nature, you can come to accept the unlimited supply of the universe. You realize you do not have to grab, fight or compete for "it" to win. Rather, what you choose and ask for, you will receive.

The complete acceptance of your Divine Nature is the foundation of knowing that you are powerful enough to attract and manifest what you want and that you are capable of successfully creating what you desire. To acknowledge and embody your divinity is to let go of all sense of abandonment that may have been instilled by your parents, friends, and society. Accepting your divinity ultimately means cutting through every illusory belief you hold that you are powerless, unworthy, limited, or forgotten, and to rest within the core (or center) of your Being. Here lies your True Nature. And it is your True Nature that shall set you free.

Card for the Day

If you were guided to this symbol today it is time to let go of all beliefs that you are less than divine. Your worthiness as a child of the universe exceeds any measure of value by man. The world is full of fear-based notions, continually reinforced in books and on TV, which promote the view that you are worthless and undesirable unless you own a myriad of material goods, or until you reach a certain status level. Reject these illusory beliefs for what they are. Choose to leave behind all feelings of unworthiness, abandonment, powerlessness or limitation. Your Divine Grandeur does not diminish with age. Accept the truth of your soul that your greatness exceeds the brightest star.

Meditation:

In a quiet space, study this symbol card and attune to its energetic essence. Feel yourself connect with the Source of your Being, and hold the symbol card up to your heart. With the symbol facing your body, ask the following, *"Beloved Divine Self, I ask that the clearest and purest energies of this symbol be infused and integrated within my Being. I now fully accept my divinity and choose that any beliefs or feelings in resistance to this truth be cleared forever from my mental, emotional, etheric and physical bodies. So be it. And so it is!'*

Visualize the sky blue color of the symbol flowing from the card into your heart and through your entire body. Allow any blocks or resistance to be flushed away by the sky blue light. Acknowledge your divinity. Sink deep into the acceptance of yourself as you might sink into a comfortable chair.

Color and Symbol Balancing

Sky blue is the symbol's primary color. The color resonates with the Love-Wisdom Ray, the second ray of the seven rays that are woven into all of creation. Blue assists in clarification because of its high vibrancy.

Gold, the symbol's secondary color, is aligned with the Christ-Ray and one's Divine Essence as a Christ Being.

Purple, the symbol's tertiary color, initiates deep purification and clearing and helps you come into alignment with Source.

Sky blue is the first recommended color to use when projecting the symbol to assist another. Visualize and feel the symbol's frequency carried on a ray of blue light. Imagine the blue color being carried throughout the entire body. When it feels as if the sky blue color has been accepted on all levels, project the symbol on a stream of gold light.

Visualize the gold light entering the heart and radiating out through the body and aura. If there appears to be resistance to accepting the symbol's essence, follow the Gold Ray with the Purple Ray. See the symbol's vibration carried on a current of rich purple light, flowing through every organ and tissue, melting away all resistance and inertia.

CARD #3

I Am Totally and Completely Protected

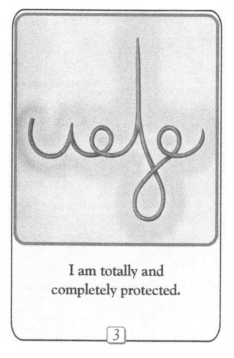

I am totally and
completely protected.

3

AFFIRMATION:

*"As I align with the Oneness of Source, I am cleared
of all opposing energies."*

Insight

This symbol helps to align you with the Source of your Being. Through this alignment you begin to carry frequencies of Light which can dissipate disruptive forces.

There is a Universal law that the higher spiritual frequencies of love and At-One-Ment (the Christ frequencies) entrain the lower frequency emotions of fear or anger and transmute them. The energy of love, being the matrix of the universe, is

CORRESPONDENCES	
PRIMARY COLOR	Electric Blue
SECONDARY COLOR	Yellow
TERTIARY COLOR	Red
METALS\CRYSTALS USED IN GRIDS:	Red Azurite\Malachite
	Blue Tourmaline
	Blue Topaz
	Blue Kyanite
	Aqua Aura
CHAKRAS CLEARED AND ALIGNED:	Throat Chakra
	Solar Plexus Chakra
MERIDIANS CLEARED AND ALIGNED:	Large Intestine Meridian
	Spleen Meridian
	Kidney Meridian
	Triple Warmer Meridian
	Gall Bladder Meridian
	Liver Meridian
PRIMARY ELEMENTS REPRESENTED BY THE SYMBOL:	Air/Fire/Water/Earth

ultimately more persuasive than fear. The more you can love and honor yourself, the easier it is to remain un-hooked from another's scripts predicated on separation.

The Divine Self's sense of protection differs from that of the ego. The ego perceives protection in terms of defense. It creates shields, barriers and walls around itself for protection, as when emotional armor is created around the heart because of past trauma.

Higher walls, bigger guns, counter-attack strategies are the kinds of protective measures undertaken by the ego-self. However, these are really acts of limitation which hinder your ability to love and to be loved, and in turn curtail your freedom.

If you operate from a belief that you are separate from others, life and Source, then enemies and arch-villains abound.

Energizing the belief that there are forces "out to get you" attracts them to you for resolution. As long as you believe there is an enemy to be fought, there will be one at your doorstep. What you resist, perpetually subsists.

The Divine Self perceives protection in terms of rising above the illusion of separation and the polarities of good and evil. When you walk in the Presence of the One, you can see and feel the fabric of unity beneath the play of the five senses.

In this state of grace and knowing, past emotional issues dissolve, "buttons" that used to be pushed disappear, and those you thought of as enemies become friends. The struggle falls away.

The most influential spiritual healers on the planet do not place shields around themselves when they work with a client. Just the opposite, they remain open and vulnerable. They allow their personal energy field to merge with those they are helping. They hold the space of love without conditions, allowing their hearts to fully embrace the client.

When they sense what are called negative emotions (anger, guilt, etc.) being released by the client in the healing session, they silently recognize that these feelings are not theirs and let them pass out of their bodies as transmuted energy without becoming attached to them.

When you can hold to your Divine Center, the Source of your Being, and know what that essence feels like, you can then distinguish your emotions from another's. And you can remain open and loving to others in your life. If you feel fear or separation from another, you can allow that emotional energy to flow through you. Your protection lies in no longer agreeing to support fear within yourself.

Card for the Day

If you were guided to select this symbol, you may be feeling that your defenses are down. At this moment you have an opportunity to muster infinite inner strength by aligning with the Divine Source of your Being. The love, wisdom and power of the universe lies within.

When you turn within and center yourself in your Divine Core, then strength, courage, and stability return. Sink deep into the unity of your Being, and the sense of separation in the outer world will evaporate.

Meditation

Study the symbol card and tune in to the energy and essence of the symbol. In a quiet space, hold the symbol card to your heart (symbol facing your body) and ask your Divine Self, *"Beloved Divine Self, I choose to embody the clearest and purest essence of this symbol within my Being. I choose to align with my Divine Core Essence and clear all fears and sense of separation from all levels of my Being. I now ask that the infinite strength, power, love and wisdom of the universe flow through me. So be it. And so it is!"*

Visualize the electric blue color of the symbol flowing into your body and up and down your spine. Imagine a blue cord of light running from the top of your head to the Central Sun in the center of the universe. See another cord of blue light running from the base of your spine into the core of the Earth.

As you inhale, draw electric blue light from the Central Sun down to your heart. And as you exhale, direct the blue light from your heart into the Earth. Cycle the electric blue light through you, using your breath, a minimum of 3 times. Meditate for a few minutes in the glow of blue light, feeling the protective quality that is created by your alignment with your Divine Core Essence.

Color and Symbolic Balancing

Electric blue, the color associated with Archangel Michael, is the primary color of this symbol. Historically electric blue is described as the color Archangel Michael uses to cut through illusion. It has a strong purifying and cleansing quality, and it helps to open the throat.

Yellow, the symbol's secondary color, assists in mental clarity and activity. It also helps to expand and clear the solar plexus chakra. Red, the tertiary color of the symbol, opens the root chakra and helps you release old emotions, such as fear and anger, into the Earth.

If the person you are working with appears ungrounded and frazzled, begin projecting the symbol on the Red Ray. Visualize the symbol's essence carried on a stream of red light that enters the root or base chakra. Allow the root chakra to expand, then see a cord of red light running from the root chakra to the core of the Earth. Silently set the intention that all the emotional complexes of separation will be grounded and released into the Earth.

Yellow helps to clear emotional issues held in the solar plexus. Visualize the symbol's energy carried on the Yellow Ray, infusing and expanding the solar plexus. Choose that all blocks in the solar plexus be dissolved by the yellow light.

After red and yellow are used to open the lower chakras, the primary color, electric blue, is recommended. Make the intention that the symbol's energy be carried within the Electric Blue Ray and project this color throughout the physical body, seeing the color expand out into the aura. Choose and see the high voltage Electric Blue Ray sweeping through every tissue, transmuting every belief and emotion based on separation into love.

CARD #4
All Life Is One

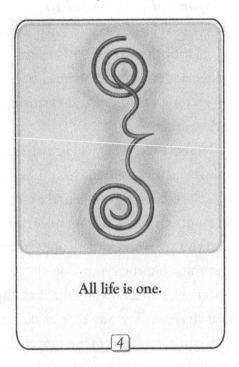

All life is one.

4

AFFIRMATION:

"All life is an expression of God. Being an extension of all life, I am supported by all life."

Insight

This symbol represents the unity of all life upon Earth. Perceiving the truth that "All Life is One," you respond by moving into harmony and balance with Nature, and life begins supporting you in ways that seem miraculous to those who perceive the world in separation.

Invisible threads of energy, light, and consciousness interconnect all life on Earth. The tapestry of life is dynamic and diverse,

CORRESPONDENCES

PRIMARY COLOR	Cobalt Blue
SECONDARY COLOR	Soft Green
TERTIARY COLOR	Bright Yellow
METALS\CRYSTALS USED IN GRIDS:	Lapis Lazuli
	Azurite
	Sodalite
	Emerald
	Peridot
CHAKRAS CLEARED AND ALIGNED:	Brow Chakra
	Throat Chakra
	Heart Chakra
	Solar Plexus Chakra
MERIDIANS CLEARED AND ALIGNED:	Stomach Meridian
	Heart Meridian
	Triple Warmer Meridian
	Liver Meridian
PRIMARY ELEMENTS REPRESENTED BY THE SYMBOL:	Earth/Fire/Water

yet, as the science of ecology has proven, the complex interplay of humans, animals and plants acts like a large living organism: breathing, growing and playing. Each human, animal, and plant is part of the flow of life, vibrantly expressing itself on a planet which is moving thousands of miles per second through the void of space. Looking at the bright blue-green jewel that is the Earth from the depths of space, it is obvious that all life is bonded as one upon her.

The essence of this symbol is about being in harmony with Nature and feeling unity with all life. When you sense the presence of this support, you realize there is permission to connect with Nature telepathically. You understand the potential of being in co-creative partnership with Nature. Through this cooperative process, dreams can more rapidly manifest and life is filled with grace.

The worldly perspective, since the dawn of the industrial and technological age, has been that mankind is separate from and in competition with Nature. Humankind, in large, has believed that natural forces needed to be overcome, tamed and subdued. Nature has been viewed as an adversary to be dealt with by force. It is logical that pollution, destruction of the rain forests, and the death of oceans, could potentially result from such a separative belief system. When it is truly understood that "**All Life is One**," and that Nature is our life support system, the rape of the planet will no longer be allowed.

This card also refers to unity of life among the human species. If you feel separate from another because of emotions like anger, fear, or pain, you have forgotten your connection with them through the life force you share. Each of us are like cells in the larger body of Earth, joyfully involved in the dance of life. Standing back and seeing the whole can assist in healing feelings of separation.

Card for the Day

If your soul guided you to this card, it is a strong suggestion to see the whole rather than the parts, to step back and sense the monumental life force coursing through the forests, seas, and cities, to feel your connection with all of life and the planet itself. It is often easier to do this kind of expansion in a natural setting. Take the time to lean against a tree, feel yourself breathing in its life force, and sense your unity with the tree.

Once you can feel your oneness with a part, expand your sphere of awareness to embody more of the whole, such as a forest, a mountain or an ocean. If you allow your expansion of awareness to grow, your perception will eventually embrace the Earth as one life, as **One Consciousness**.

Meditation

In a secluded spot, study the symbol, its energy and essence. Bring the symbol to your heart (symbol facing your body) and ask, *"Beloved Divine Self, I choose to embody the highest qualities and vibrations of this symbol and to perceive "All Life As One." I also choose that all resistance and inertia to this intention be cleared and transformed to unity and love. So be it. And so it is."*

As you breathe, draw the cobalt blue color of the symbol into your heart and allow the color to flow through your entire body. Choose to come into resonance with all life on Mother Earth, and sink into the feeling of unity that naturally exists within the planet.

Color and Symbol Balancing

Cobalt blue, the symbol's primary color, is the ray most strongly associated with Earth. It has protective qualities, shielding you against disruptive energies.

Green, the symbol's secondary color, is another color which resonates with the Earth as well as the heart. Green helps to open the heart chakra and balances the physical body, bringing it into alignment with the planet.

Yellow, the symbol's tertiary color, helps to clarify the mental body and open the solar plexus chakra, allowing you to be more centered and grounded.

Use cobalt blue when broadcasting the symbol's frequency to someone. Imagine the symbol's essence carried on a stream of cobalt blue light. Visualize the cobalt blue light sweeping through the body from head to foot, clearing away any resistance to the symbol's vibration. Imagine the cobalt blue light flowing down from the recipient's feet into the center of Earth, solidly grounding them into the planet.

Follow cobalt blue with the Green Ray. See and feel the symbol's energy carried on a current of soft green light. Visualize the soft green light entering the heart, then radiating through the entire body. As you do this, set the intention that the cellular memory of the individual resonate with the truth *"that all life is one and that you are one with all life."*

If the solar plexus appears to be blocked, broadcast the symbol on the Yellow Ray, visualizing the solar plexus infused with radiant yellow and all darkness transmuted to light. Then follow with the Cobalt Blue and Green Rays.

CARD #5

I Now Clear All Pain and Sense of Separation

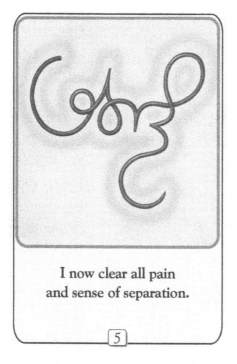

I now clear all pain
and sense of separation.

5

AFFIRMATION

"I realize that I have never been separate and I surrender to the unity which is the foundation of my being."

Insight

This symbol supports the feeling of connection, safety, peace, and well being, the sense that you are already Home. Separation from Source, others and Self is an illusion. You have never been separate. However, you can live in a bubble of beliefs that you are isolated, alone and disconnected. As long as you subscribe to those beliefs, you will emotionally experience the pain of separation.

CORRESPONDENCES

PRIMARY COLOR	Royal Purple
SECONDARY COLOR	Soft Green
TERTIARY COLOR	Electric Blue
METALS\CRYSTALS USED IN GRIDS:	Sugilite-Luvulite
	Purple/violet Fluorite
	Azurite
	Purpurite
CHAKRAS CLEARED AND ALIGNED:	Crown Chakra
	Brow Chakra
	Throat Chakra
MERIDIANS CLEARED AND ALIGNED:	Small Intestine Meridian
	Pericardium Meridian
	Triple Warmer Meridian
PRIMARY ELEMENTS REPRESENTED BY THE SYMBOL:	Ether/Air/Fire

The last thing a fish discovers is water because it is fully immersed within it. If you are immersed in the thought-forms of separation, you can only extricate yourself through the choice to do so.

Many of the mass consciousness beliefs surrounding separation are predicated on the assumption that you are no more than a physical body. If you choose to believe you are only your physical body, and remain emotionally attached to the form, pain is sure to arise when the form changes. In truth, you are so much more. You are an extension of the Universal Field, which is infinite in nature.

The belief system of separation is perpetuated every time you feel you are unworthy, that you aren't good enough, or that you lack something. And when you see yourself or someone else as less than divine, you further energize the collective beliefs supporting the illusion of separation.

It takes tremendous energy to maintain our illusory barriers. The energy locked in the bubble of separation can begin to be transmuted once you embody the understanding that you are **One** and that what appears to be fragmented is really whole and complete.

Perhaps the reason we experience isolation is to discover *"this is not where it's at,"* thus creating an opportunity to choose love instead.

I suspect that a part of the pain of separation arises from the inner knowing, at the core of our being, that we could live in love and unity rather than in isolation. The pain experienced points to another path filled with joy. Countless books have discussed how to move beyond separation. Summarizing their wisdom, these basic steps are suggested:

1. First, acknowledge any feelings of anger, fear, hate, jealousy, and guilt, as old emotional programs that don't support your sense of unity. As you feel these old energies, choose to let them go forever.

2. Choose to see the unity and divinity in all things. When you can see Source in others, you can see Source within yourself.

3. Refuse to judge, blame, criticize, or even hold opinions, of others. Any kind of emotional judgment of another perpetuates the illusion of separation within yourself and, in turn, the collective consciousness.

4. Embrace any fear, anger, or pain with love. Choose to see the holiness of all life. Communicate to everyone and every thing in your life its sacredness and it will become

that in your eyes.

Card for the Day

If you were guided to this symbol today it is time to let go and let love flow into your life. It is far more joyful to feel your unity with others than to feel cut off and separate from them.

If you are experiencing a sense of separation from someone or some thing, the following meditation is recommended.

Meditation

In a quiet location, study the symbol's form and color. Hold the symbol card to your heart chakra (the symbol facing your body) and ask, "*Beloved Divine Self, I choose to embody the highest qualities of this symbol. I now dissolve all feelings and beliefs in separation from self, others and Source. I choose that these old energies be transmuted to love—now and forever. So be it. And so it is.*"

Feel the symbol's purple color flow into your heart and your body, sweeping out old energies and beliefs. Allow the symbol's vibration and deep purple light to dissolve and clear any constrictions or tightness you may feel.

The visualization exercise described for symbol *Card #8, "I am loved. I love. I am love."* is also recommended. Visualize reconnecting with the person or object you feel disconnected from; use the energy of love from your heart to reunite yourself with that individual or object.

Color and Symbol Balancing

Royal purple is the symbol's primary color. Purple aligns you on the core level with your spiritual essence. It also helps purify discordant energies not in alignment with the *Truth of your Being.*

Green, the symbol's secondary color, assists the physical body in reaching balance, harmony, and peace. Green works through the heart chakra, achieving balance in sky and Earth energies (the up-flowing and down-flowing energies within the body).

Electric blue, the symbol's tertiary color, resonates with the blue of Archangel Michael's Ray and helps cut through blockages created by fear and belief in separation.

Electric blue is recommended as the first color to use when broadcasting the vibration of this symbol to someone. Visualize the symbol's energy carried on a stream of electric blue light, moving through the entire body. Imagine the blue light filled with small flecks of white light that brightly sparkle and dissolve away any blocks held in the chakras and body tissues.

After it feels like the blockages have been cleared, project the symbol's vibration on a current of purple light. See rich purple light filling each chakra and the entire spine, flowing out into all the organs and tissues to assist the physical body in reaching balance.

Complete the *light work* by broadcasting the symbol on the Green Ray. Infuse the heart chakra with green light, seeing it radiate out from the heart and through the whole being.

CARD #6

I Trust and Follow My Heart

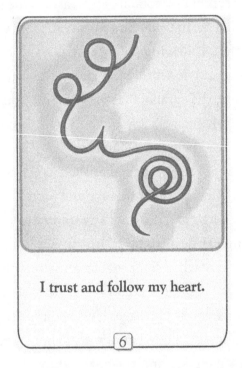

I trust and follow my heart.

6

AFFIRMATION

"I Listen to my heart for guidance and walk my path in love."

Insight

This symbol supports one walking daily in the space of love. Trusting love in your life is being open to the full exchange of resources and opportunities that result from loving yourself, others, and all that you do. Yet the left brain may perceive that what the heart wants to do is foolish, for it has difficulty understanding the rationale of *"love."*

Feeling and being loving is non-linear, expansive, and opens

CORRESPONDENCES

PRIMARY COLOR	Pink
SECONDARY COLOR	Bright Lemon Yellow
TERTIARY COLOR	Gold
METALS\CRYSTALS USED IN GRIDS:	Rose Quartz
	Pink Kunzite
	Gold Citrine
	Gold Topaz
CHAKRAS CLEARED AND ALIGNED:	Heart Chakra
	Solar Plexus Chakra
	Root Chakra
MERIDIANS CLEARED AND ALIGNED:	Spleen Meridian
	Heart Meridian
	Kidney Meridian
	Gall Bladder Meridian
	Liver Meridian
PRIMARY ELEMENTS REPRESENTED BY THE SYMBOL:	Fire/Earth/Water

you to infinite growth. The infinite Universal Flow that you access through love is beyond the grasp of all analytical paradigms. Cost/benefit ratios, spread-sheet analyses, "good versus bad" are left brain concepts that have to be set aside if you are going to ask your heart for direction, for the heart is guided by love.

You move through various cycles in your life. Some days you feel freer and more uplifted than others. You appear to cycle through periods of expansion and contraction. Fear creates the state of contraction—love manifests the state of expansion. When you are in fear, there is a tendency to withdraw and become tense. During these times, you may experience severe pain because of cramped muscles.

When you embody love, you energetically expand, becoming more flexible, feeling open and powerful. You are in the flow. One experiences increased vitality. When you trust your heart, you are on the path of joy and health. The heart chakra is the access point to the Divine Self, representing the balance of cosmic and Earth energies, the upper and lower chakras.

Following your heart is the most important step in moving away from the dominance of the ego-mind. It is a shift from a fear based perception to one of trust in the *Divine Design* and the knowing that everything is unfolding as it should. Trust and love are intimately connected.

The more heart-based your decisions, the more you can trust the flow of your life and the lessons presented. Trusting the guidance of your heart is the path of expansion and growth. It is the way of the soul. Following your heart involves down-playing the divisions and limitations of the mind. It involves accepting your own innate and Divine Nature, and loving yourself so fully there remains no room for fear.

Card for the Day

If this card is chosen, you may have opportunities arising to move into a more expanded state of love and trust. Your Divine Self is suggesting it is time to shift your attention away from your mind to your heart. The guidance from your heart will move you into expansion and grace. The following meditation is recommended.

Meditation

In a peaceful space, study the symbol, its form, shape and color. Then hold the symbol card to your heart (symbol facing your body). Ask your Divine Self, "*Beloved, Divine Self, I choose to now absorb the purest and most loving energies of this symbol into my heart, body and Being. I choose to listen to my heart for*

*guidance and to be shown the path of greatest joy in my life. I
ask that this be done now. So be it. And so it is."*

Visualize pink light from the symbol card carrying the energy
of the symbol into your heart. Feel the essence of the symbol flow
through your body and being. Allow images of the next steps
of action to enter your mind's eye as you stay centered in your
heart. What course of action expands the heart to the greatest
degree? Allow your heart to show you the way.

Color and Symbol Balancing

Pink is the primary color of this symbol. Pink helps expand
self-love and fosters acceptance of love in your life.

Bright lemon, the symbol's secondary color, embodies the
green and yellow colors in approximately equal proportions. The
green aspect enhances clearing and balance, helping to open the
heart chakra. The yellow aspect assists in the purification of the
solar plexus chakra and the expansion of your personal power.

Gold, the symbol's tertiary color, is the color of the Christ
Ray. It aligns you to your soul essence.

When projecting the symbol's energy toward someone, it is
recommended to first use the Gold and Lemon Rays. Visualize
lemon and gold light carrying the symbol's vibration, entering
the solar plexus and expanding out through the body, burning
away all darkness and blocks. When it feels that all resistance
has been cleared, begin broadcasting the symbol's frequency on
a current of pink light.

Allow the pink light to fill the heart and expand out through
the chest, solar plexus, head, arms and legs. See the entire body
radiating glorious pink light. Affirm that the individual trusts
and follows his/her heart in all ways.

CARD #7

I Look Within for Divine Wisdom

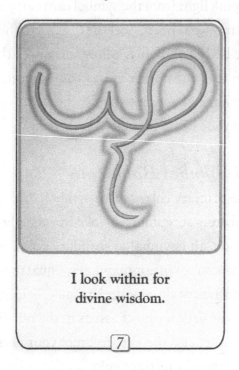

I look within for
divine wisdom.

7

AFFIRMATION

"I know all the answers I need lie within me and I now go within to contact the wisdom of the universe."

Insight

All the knowledge and wisdom of the universe is held within yourself. You need only look to your soul essence to find the answers for which you are searching. However you must first turn within and ask.

We are acculturated by our society to believe that people, institutions, and organizations hold all the answers. If you come from a belief that the wisdom you need is outside of you, you

CORRESPONDENCES	
PRIMARY COLOR	Dark Blue
SECONDARY COLOR	Light Blue
TERTIARY COLOR	Peach Pink
METALS\CRYSTALS USED IN GRIDS:	Lapis Lazuli
	Azurite/Malachite
	Labradorite
	Blue Sapphire
	Sodalite
CHAKRAS CLEARED AND ALIGNED:	Brow Chakra
	Throat Chakra
MERIDIANS CLEARED AND ALIGNED:	Urinary Bladder Meridian
	Triple Warmer Meridian
	Gall Bladder Meridian
PRIMARY ELEMENTS REPRESENTED BY THE SYMBOL:	Air/Fire/Water

have divorced yourself from your own magnificence.

You are an extension of a holographic universe. And in the same way that each small part of a hologram carries the information of the entire hologram, you are linked through resonance to the wisdom contained in the entire Universal Field.

Accessing the source of Divine Wisdom within involves cultivating a dialogue with your Divine Self, asking and listening for answers from your Soul Essence, and taking the time to listen to the still voice within. This is a natural and easy process, as easy as laughing at a good joke. It only appears difficult when it has not been practiced. Just like learning to ride a bike, turning within for guidance becomes second nature with practice.

The Divine Guidance received from your soul can differ from the wisdom of the world. The soul is concerned with the primary spiritual focus of "How deeply do you love yourself, love others, and love Source?" From this vantage point, the guidance from your soul may seem to counter the prevalent world-view.

For example, your soul might determine that if you helped a village in Africa, your ability to love and be loved would grow at a much faster rate than working as a Wall Street banker, and in turn might guide you to take a Peace Corps job. The world-view would be that you would be more economically secure as a banker.

If you were strongly invested in the viewpoint that your worth is measured by financial income, your beliefs could act as a filter, blocking the guidance of the voice within. Humbly quieting your mind and accepting your soul's wisdom, even if it runs counter to the world-view, enhances your receptivity.

The more you turn within for Universal wisdom, the easier the guidance will come to you. In time, you need not ask the question, for the answer appears before it is posed. At that point, you will have stepped into the Universal Flow, allowing your Divine Nature to guide your life.

Card for the Day

If you have selected this card, you very likely have a question or issue in your life that your soul wants to assist you with.

The wisdom, understanding, and solution to the issue lies within you. Deep within the Core of Your Being exists the answers to all the questions you could ask. Indeed, you carry the wisdom of the ages within you. It may be temporarily masked by the hustle and bustle of daily life, but after the surface confusion is cleared, the deep well of Universal wisdom can be found.

Meditation

Choose a quiet place and time to go within your heart, connect to your soul, and ask for a solution that's in your highest good. Allow yourself to be open to guidance even though it may appear illogical. Your soul may answer you in unexpected ways (through dreams, comments made by chance encounters, messages over the radio, or even statements made on personal license plates). Be open to receive the messages, either now or in the coming days, and joyfully await your answer.

Color and Symbol Balancing

Dark blue, the primary color of the symbol, helps to activate the Brow Chakra.

The symbol's secondary color, light blue, helps expand the throat chakra, assisting you to walk your talk and creatively express your mission.

Peach pink, the symbol's tertiary color, resonates with the heart chakra and the love vibration.

It is recommended that you first project the symbol's vibration to the heart chakra of the recipient on a current of peach pink light. Visualize the heart chakra filled to over-flowing with the peach pink light.

Then move up to the throat, projecting the symbol's frequency on a stream of light blue light and infusing the throat chakra.

Finally, move up to the Brow Chakra and project dark blue along with the symbol's essence into the Brow Chakra. Affirm that the wisdom of the universe is accessible to the individual.

CARD #8

I Am Loved. I Love. I Am Love.

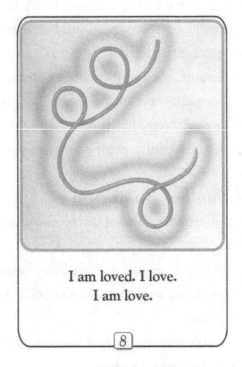

I am loved. I love.
I am love.

8

AFFIRMATION

"I see myself and all in my life as worthy of love and lovable. I love others as I choose to be loved."

Insight

This symbol carries the essence of the Second Ray, the Universal Ray of Divine Love. It is the love that binds the stars and galaxies, it exists beyond form and within form. The symbol embodies the quality of loving and being loved simply because you exist, not for what you do or what you own.

When you hold this state of consciousness, you bring its universal nature into the physical and create the space for others in

CORRESPONDENCES	
Primary Color	Gold
Secondary Color	Pinkish Red
Tertiary Color	Silver
Metals\Crystals Used In Grids:	Gold Topaz
	Gold (metal)
	Pink Kunzite
	Pink Tourmaline
	Rose Quartz
	Rhodachrosite
	Lepidolite with Pink Tourmaline
	Watermelon Tourmaline
Chakras Cleared and Aligned:	Heart Chakra
	Root Chakra
Meridians Cleared and Aligned:	Heart Meridian
	Urinary Bladder Meridian
	Kidney Meridian
Primary Elements Represented by the Symbol:	Water/Fire/Earth

your life to love themselves.

Perhaps your greatest soul lesson is to learn to love all aspects of yourself, to love away all the judgments you have placed upon yourself and others. It involves a shift in perception from seeing self and others as less than, lacking, unworthy, or wrong, to seeing them as divine, worthy, and lovable.

The subconscious records all your judgments of others, and will mirror those judgments back. If, for example, you feel you are overweight and at the same time judge others as less than desirable because they are fat, your subconscious will turn these same judgments inward to poison your own self image. The way out, of course, is to stop judging. Love and accept others in the same way you would want to be loved. It involves seeing beyond the surface to the very core of their being, which remains Divine.

When you perceive and judge inconsistencies in others, you reinforce their dysfunctional image of themselves which they have projected into the world, thus supporting the continuation of those beliefs and patterns.

However, when you see through the surface to their core essence of divinity and love them for who they truly are, a paradigm of wholeness is reinforced and allowed to manifest in their lives. As you love others for their Divine Nature, they will begin to love and honor themselves.

Love without conditions is an energetic frequency within the Universal Field of which you are a part. When you choose to perceive another as lovable, that energy is conveyed via resonance through the Universal Field to the person. The recipient will feel the love on a subconscious level, although they may not actually perceive it consciously. Nevertheless, love is transferred and experienced.

Love is the most potent healing force on the planet, even when it's conveyed at a distance. It clears the lower vibratory emotions of anger, fear, guilt, and shame. It heals through all energy bodies (spiritual, mental, emotional, etheric, and physical) to bring balance and harmony to the individual. True healing can only be accomplished through self-acceptance and self-love. Indeed, there is nothing more powerful or unifying than love fully expressed.

Card for the Day

If your Divine Self guided you to this card, it is an important time to bring more love into your life, and to see yourself as worthy of love. The following meditation is recommended if you are feeling separate from someone or some thing (e.g., financial abundance).

Meditation

Study the symbol card and relax into its energy. Hold the symbol card to your heart (symbol facing your body) and request, *"Beloved, Divine Self, I choose to now embody the highest essence of Divine Love in my life, and to transmute any sense of separation. So be it. And so it is."*

Visualize the pink color of the symbol flowing into your heart, allowing your heart to soften and expand. When your heart feels open, see before you the person or thing you feel separate from. Ask to draw in the unconditional and Divine Love of the universe. Visualize a current of pink light entering your crown as you inhale. When you exhale, imagine a beam of pink light leaving your heart and connecting with the person or thing from which you feel separate.

Now, create a loop of pink light. As you inhale, draw pink light from the person or thing; and as you exhale, project a current of pink light in return until the sense of separation lessens. As the feeling of separation diminishes, see the person or thing move towards you. Then see, sense, and feel the person or thing merge with you.

In some cases, the sense of separation can run very deep and you may have to repeat this meditation a number of times to clear the emotional charges.

Color and Symbol Balancing

The primary color of this symbol is gold, aligned with the

Christos and the vibration of unconditional love.

Pinkish red, the secondary color, activates the heart as well as the root chakra and resonates with the love of the Divine Mother.

Silver, the tertiary color, is the ray of the Divine Feminine—acceptance and allowance.

When projecting the symbol's energy toward someone, it is recommended that you first project the symbol's essence on the Pinkish-Red Ray. Imagine the pinkish-red light entering the heart and see the heart unfolding and blossoming like a rose. This color will assist in grounding the vibration of love into the physical. Visualize the pinkish-red light surrounding the heart and flowing down through the body, out the feet into the Earth. Hold this visualization until it feels like it has "*locked in.*"

Follow this visualization by projecting the symbol on the Gold Christ Ray. See a current of gold light flowing through and filling the body. Visualize the gold light radiating out through the body into space. Imagine the body radiant, washed in golden light.

If the person appears ungrounded or scattered, use the light of the Silver Ray before broadcasting the Pinkish-Red or Gold Ray. See silver light carrying the symbol's vibration flowing through the left side of the body and through the three lower chakras (root, sexual, and solar plexus). As you do this, hold the intention that the muscles relax and that the tension is dissolved.

CARD #9

I Transmute All Pain to Love.

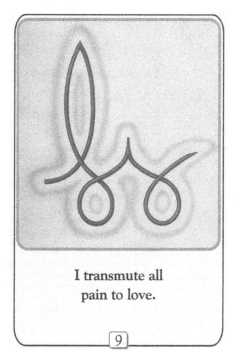

I transmute all
pain to love.

9

AFFIRMATION

"As I love, all pain created through separation is transmuted."

Insight

Most pain arises from a mental and emotional state of separation. It dissolves when you allow the unity of love to be felt. The universe is held together by the continual exchange of energy (love) between all aspects of Source. Any attempt to separate from this exchange of energy (love) is illusory and painful. Pain manifests when mental and emotional energy is expended to create walls and barriers to the eternally-present Universal Love.

Correspondences

Primary Color	Purple
Secondary Color	Pink
Tertiary Color	Gold
Metals\Crystals Used In Grids:	Amethyst
	Sugilite–Luvulite
	Violet Fluorite
	Rose Quartz
	Lepidolite with Pink Tourmaline
Chakras Cleared and Aligned:	Crown Chakra
	Throat Chakra
	Heart Chakra
Meridians Cleared and Aligned:	Spleen/Pancreas Meridian
	Heart Meridian
	Gall Bladder Meridian
	Liver Meridian
Primary Elements Represented by the Symbol:	Air/Fire/Earth

Emotional pain is resistance to love, and it usually arises from the internal mental conflict that results when you simultaneously hold two opposing beliefs (e.g. "*Yes, I can do it*" and "*No, I can't do it.*") Once the conflict is resolved, the pain—even if it's physical—will often immediately clear.

You usually perceive yourself in terms of your physical body. However, as an extension of the Universal Field of Source, your consciousness extends infinitely far beyond your skin. You draw choices to you through the Universal Field. In the broadest sense, nothing is outside of you, and the Source of your Being is within.

Your beliefs attract and manifest your experience. Your power lies in being fully aware of your co-creative nature and the knowledge that your "outer" world is an extension of your "inner" world.

Emotional pain is generated by the illusion that there is an external reality which can have an effect on you. This illusion is supported by the erroneous belief that your circumstances are divorced from your choices and perceptions.

Pain indicates you have given your power away, believing you are separate from the universe. This pain can be viewed as a wake-up call to the truth that you are a co-creator of your experience. You manifest what you experience. Pain demonstrates a belief in separation that holds you in isolation from the truth, from others, and from the Source of your Being.

This *Waveform Symbol* helps to clear the misperception that reality is external and separate from you. It assists in healing the illusory split from the Universal Field created by the mind. This symbol resonates with the Christos essence. It is aligned with the unifying force of love, for it is through love that the walls of fear are transmuted.

The symbol assists in shifting the focus from pain to unity and joy. Healing means to make whole again, reuniting the painful fragments you have created in your mind. It is through love that healing is accomplished and that union is experienced.

Card for the Day

If you were guided to this card, you may be experiencing pain in some part of your life. The pain suggests it is time to honor yourself, to love yourself as your best friend. Take yourself out to a movie, treat yourself to a meal at the best restaurant in town, or purchase a gift for yourself which you have always wanted to receive.

Look at yourself in a full length mirror and see yourself as the

Divine Being that you are. Identify all those qualities within your life which are positive and uplifting. Look beneath the skin and see the stardust which composes your physical form. Know that you are a unique expression of the Divine Force flowing through all things. Choose to love yourself to such a degree that all the pain you hold is transmuted. Choose to be whole and complete. As an extension of Source, you are worthy of love. So, above all else, love yourself.

Meditation

Study the form, color and essence of the symbol card. In a secluded place, hold the symbol card up to your heart (symbol facing your body) and ask, "*Beloved Divine Self, I choose that the clearest, purest, and highest transformational qualities of this symbol fill my entire being, transmuting all sense of pain and separation to love and joy. I choose this transmutation occurs now through all levels. So be it. And so it is.*"

Feel the essence of the symbol flood your body along with the color purple. Choose that any pain you are experiencing be cleared. Accept the color purple into your cells, penetrating and clearing all fear, upset, and pain.

After you sense the old emotional energies dissipating, allow pink light to fill your body and Being. Repeat the following phrase silently, "*I am okay just the way I am.*" Acknowledge from the Core of Your Being that this is true.

Color and Symbol Balancing

The primary color of the symbol is purple, the color of purification. Because of purple's high frequency, it has the ability to shift lower vibratory emotions such as fear and grief to higher frequencies of light. Purple also assists in expanding the crown chakra.

Pink, the symbol's secondary color, helps to open the heart chakra to love and acceptance. Pink is composed of the colors red and white: the red aspect assists in opening the root chakra and grounding one into life and the planet. The white aspect, composed of the seven spectrum colors, helps to open and balance the seven major chakras.

Gold, the symbol's tertiary color, is aligned to the Christos essence and one's Divine Core. The Gold Ray is purifying and resonates with the universal aspect of love.

When projecting the symbol's energy toward someone, begin by broadcasting the symbol on a current of purple light. Imagine the purple light cascading like a shower, down, over, and through the recipient, clearing any blockages held in the body or aura. Set the intention that the highest vibrations of the symbol transmute all separation and pain to love.

Once it feels as if the issues of separation have been cleared, follow with the color of pink. Visualize the symbol's frequency carried by a Ray of Pink Light which enters the heart and radiates through the entire body. See the heart chakra opening like a pink rose. Choose that the individual embodies Universal Love on all levels.

Use gold light as the final color to transmit the symbol's frequency. Visualize the Gold Ray filling and infusing all cells, tissues, and parts of the body. Silently acknowledge the person's divinity and his/her unity with all life.

CARD #10

I Accept and Receive the Manifestation of My Desire

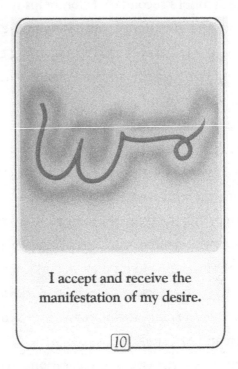

I accept and receive the
manifestation of my desire.

10

AFFIRMATION

*"I give myself permission to accept and receive my
desire and allow it to ground into form."*

Insight

It is okay to have what you want. However, you need to feel
worthy of receiving your desire. The universe has a wondrous
gift for you just outside the door, but you have to open the door
and allow it in.

You often cut yourself off from the Universal Flow by find-
ing some reason why you can't allow your desires to manifest in
your life. Perhaps you feel you can't be wealthy and spiritual at

CORRESPONDENCES

PRIMARY COLOR	Red
SECONDARY COLOR	Orange
TERTIARY COLOR	Yellow
METALS\CRYSTALS USED IN GRIDS:	Garnet
	Raw Ruby
	Red Jasper
	Carnelian
	Yellow Citrine
CHAKRAS CLEARED AND ALIGNED:	Root Chakra
	Sexual Chakra
MERIDIANS CLEARED AND ALIGNED:	Pericardium Meridian
	Spleen Meridian
PRIMARY ELEMENTS REPRESENTED BY THE SYMBOL:	Earth/Fire

the same time. Maybe you feel you can only manifest the desire in a specific way following prescribed steps. Any other way isn't allowed because you would not be in control.

Feeling you don't deserve love, abundance, or friends is a powerful way of pushing the Universal Flow away from you. Believing you are unworthy and separate from what you desire closes the door on your ability to receive it, even if it's right beside you.

Allow yourself to believe. Just say, "**Yes.**" The universe desires to give you what you want. Let go of the constricting needs of personality to control the outcome and the way your dream has to manifest.

Let go of the beliefs that you are unworthy and undeserving. You are a child of Source and of the Universe. Abundance, love, and wisdom are your natural inheritance. Anything is possible.

An important aspect of this symbol is allowing your desire

to become physical, to ground your intention into the third dimension. To do this, it helps if you are open to the feminine Earth energy. The magnetic enfolding energy of Mother Earth is necessary in manifesting your desire into physical form.

The *"I accept and receive the manifestation of my desire"* symbol activates and opens the root or base chakra, which energetically connects you to Mother Earth. The symbol assists you in embracing and allowing the feminine Earth energy into your Being.

When people feel separate from the Earth, they often "close down" their base chakra, disconnecting from Earth's magnetic field. In this state, it is much more difficult for them to create what they want. Opening the door to Universal abundance involves allowing the Earth energy to flow freely through your being.

Three symbols in the *Waveform Card Deck* focus on manifestation:

Card #10: *I accept and receive the manifestation of my desire.*

Card #30: *I welcome the manifestation of my desire.*

Card #28: *I choose the completion of my desire.*

The *"I accept and receive the manifestation of my desire"* symbol embodies the choice: *"Yes, I am worthy and deserve my desire."* It involves opening the base chakra and grounding the vision into the physical.

The *"I welcome the manifestation of my desire"* symbol opens the heart chakra and lovingly invites your desire to be with you.

The *"I choose the completion of my desire"* symbol assists you in jumping off the fence of fear and choosing to see your desire manifested. This symbol activates the solar plexus chakra and helps you take back the power that has been blocked by indecision. Each of these aspects are important if you want to joyfully and rapidly manifest your dream.

Card for the Day

If you selected this card, it is a propitious time to allow a vision, a dream, or a person to come into your life. Choose to feel worthy and deserving of your desire. Be okay with yourself in the choosing, receiving, and experiencing of your dream. Give yourself permission to have all that you desire. Allow yourself to live your greatest aspirations. Open the door to your vision and allow it into your life.

Meditation

Walk the Earth. Feel your intimate connection to Her. Allow the Earth energy to flow up your feet and legs into your whole body. As you walk the Earth and draw its magnetic essence into you, begin visualizing that your dreams have already manifested. Imagine that your wish is already fulfilled.

Allow yourself to emotionally experience the joy and thrill of the manifested desire. When the flush of excitement courses through your Being, your vision has actualized on a higher dimensional level. The blueprint has been activated and imprinted with love. Then, in the absence of fear or doubt, allow your desire to appear on Earth.

Color and Symbol Balancing

Red is the primary color of this symbol. It assists in expanding the root (base) chakra, allowing you to feel grounded, centered, and anchored in Mother Earth.

The secondary and tertiary colors of the symbol (orange and yellow) activate and open the second and third chakras (sexual and solar plexus), which are also involved in maintaining and grounding the physical body on the Earth plane.

When projecting the vibration of this symbol toward another, visualize it being carried on a current of red light. See the red light infusing the root chakra, then expanding as a cord of light traveling down to the core of the Earth, linking the individual to the core of the Earth.

If the person appears to hold fear and doubt about manifesting his or her visions, utilize the Yellow Ray to clear and open the individual's solar plexus.

Visualize the Yellow Ray carrying the frequency of the symbol, filling the solar plexus chakra with such intensity that all blockages are transmuted to brilliant yellow light.

If the individual appears to have a blocked sexual chakra or speaks of feeling joyless, then direct the energy of the symbol's Orange Ray into his or her second chakra. See and feel the sexual chakra opening and expanding.

CARD #11
I Am Aligned with My Soul's Purpose

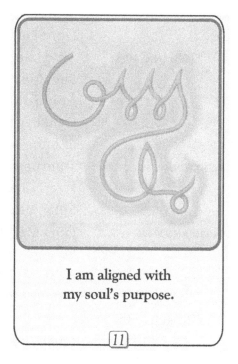

I am aligned with
my soul's purpose.

11

AFFIRMATION

*"I now dissolve all resistance to manifesting my
soul's mission."*

Insight

This symbol helps to energetically re-align your life on all
levels (relationships, job, thoughts, goals) to your soul's purpose.
It helps to open you to receiving guidance from your soul concerning your next step, and then accepting that guidance. It also
assists you in choosing to clear any inertia which is keeping you
from manifesting your highest good.

When you go deep within the Core of Your Being and medi-

CORRESPONDENCES	
PRIMARY COLOR	Gold
SECONDARY COLOR	Yellow
TERTIARY COLOR	Light Purple
METALS\CRYSTALS USED IN GRIDS:	Gold (metal)
	Sunstone-Heliolite
	Gold Rutilated Quartz
	Gold Barite
	Lithium
CHAKRAS CLEARED AND ALIGNED:	Transpersonal Chakra
	Heart Chakra
	Solar Plexus Chakra
MERIDIANS CLEARED AND ALIGNED:	Lung Meridian
	Spleen Meridian
	Heart Meridian
	Kidney Meridian
PRIMARY ELEMENTS REPRESENTED BY THE SYMBOL:	Ether/Fire/Earth/Water

tate on your life, often a sense of knowing wells up, reminding you that you are here for a special purpose. Usually this has nothing to do with the guidelines presented to you by society. For example, it is most likely not about making a lot of money, acquiring status symbols, accumulating sexual conquests, or becoming famous for the sake of power. You may have chosen on a soul level to clear all anger and to live a life of forgiveness, to raise a child in the space of unconditional love, or to be of service to others in their spiritual growth.

There is a simple way to tell whether or not you are aligned with what your soul chose to accomplish. If your life makes your heart sing and fills you with joy, chances are good that you are in alignment with your soul's purpose. If, however, you find your job dull and boring, you often feel depressed, or have low vitality, then you are very likely out of alignment with your soul's guidance.

The spiritual energy flooding the planet is growing more intense every day; it is awakening and reminding everyone to manifest their life's purpose. With each passing year, it will prove more difficult to resist the call of your soul to be all you can be. Resistance will only create inner conflict and pain. Should you heed the calls of your Divine Self and express your Core Soul mission, your joy will be beyond measure. Your life will ripen with meaning and laughter, and you will feel yourself in the Universal Flow.

There is no need to fret if you don't consciously know your soul's path. Your heart knows the way. Listen to its song. Do what feels right in your heart. Say what your heart wants to express. If you appear to be at a crossroads, review your options and then make the choice to walk the path that expands your heart.

Our soul's mission to fully express the love of Source can be reached successfully only through the way of the heart. The mind with its logic, analytical reasoning, and discriminating theories cannot be the well-spring for Divine Love. The heart is the fountainhead for the love of Source, love of self, and love of another. Use your heart as a guide, for it knows your soul's purpose well and will lead you on a true course.

Card for the Day

If you are guided to select this card, you are at an auspicious point and have a chance to more closely align with your soul's purpose. It is an opportunity to walk the path filled with the greatest joy. Look at the options you have available and step into each one. Imagine yourself fully immersed in its energy.

What does the option feel like? Does your heart expand or contract? Does your body energetically feel depleted or does it seem like you have boundless energy? Choose the option that fills your heart, makes you smile, and allows energy to course through you. You have just chosen your soul's path.

Meditation

Should the path be unclear, prayer is a powerful and wonderful way to address your soul with questions. Sit in meditation. Bring your focus to your heart and visualize it as a doorway to your soul essence. Imagine yourself moving through a heart doorway and connecting with your soul energy. Make the following request, *"Beloved Divine Self, show me the next step to take that is in alignment with my highest good. I choose to clear all resistance to the complete manifestation of my soul's mission now. So be it. And so it is."*

Relax and allow the answer to flow in. Often, putting this request to your soul just before going to sleep results in answers in the form of dreams.

Color and Symbol Balancing

The Gold Christ Ray is the primary color of this symbol. It resonates strongly with one's soul essence. The Gold Ray activates the heart chakra, as well as chakras above the head. It also expands the energy in the lungs and the physical heart.

Visualize the Gold Ray filling the heart area, the lungs, and then flowing through the whole body. Choose, as the organs and chakras fill with gold light, that they become aligned with the individual's highest good.

Yellow, the secondary color of this symbol helps open and energize the solar plexus chakra, allowing the Gold Christ Ray to be grounded into the physical and emotional bodies.

Project the vibration of this symbol on gold and yellow currents of Light. Visualize the yellow light filling the solar plexus, expanding and clearing any darkness present. See the gold light filling the heart area.

As the final step, see a gold column of light running from the Great Central Sun, flowing down the spine, and into the core of the Earth. (See *The Sacred Core Visualization*, pages 45-46.)

CARD #12

I Am Free

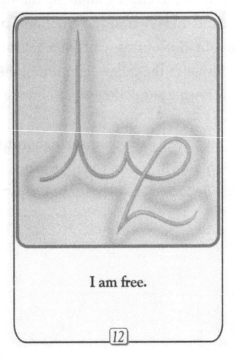

I am free.

12

AFFIRMATION

"I free myself of the bondage and barriers of judgement and fear created by myself."

Insight

When you feel separate from others and the world, you place barriers around yourself which limit your freedom. Judgments about yourself and others, such as anger, jealousy, fear, create invisible chasms between you and the ones you have judged. Your freedom is reduced because you have chosen to limit your response in a prescribed way. Judgment creates bondage.

Freedom, in turn, arises from forgiveness and from letting

CORRESPONDENCES	
PRIMARY COLOR	Bright Yellow
SECONDARY COLOR	Salmon Pink
TERTIARY COLOR	Red
METALS\CRYSTALS USED IN GRIDS:	Yellow Citrine
	Yellow Tiger Eye
	Yellow Garnet
	Yellow Amber
	Sunstone–Heliolite
	Peach Aventurine
CHAKRAS CLEARED AND ALIGNED:	Solar Plexus Chakra
	Sexual Chakra
MERIDIANS CLEARED AND ALIGNED:	Large Intestine Meridian
	Small Intestine Meridian
	Kidney Meridian
	Pericardium Meridian
PRIMARY ELEMENTS REPRESENTED BY THE SYMBOL:	Ether/Fire/Water/Earth

go of the need to be right.

Fear is the greatest slayer of freedom. Many people feeling fear perceive it as an impassable wall and move no further to pursue their dream. Freedom results from having the courage to feel the fear, move through it, and take an action step, start the project, or make the commitment, regardless. After taking the action step(s) you discover that your fears, which felt so solid, dissolve into wispy smoke. The courage to face your greatest fears is the gateway to your unlimited freedom.

One of the powerful brakes you place on yourself is worrying about what others might think if you did something unconventional. Freedom lies in being true to your Core Essence by listening to your small inner voice and following its guidance. Freedom is heeding the direction of your soul above logic. It's trusting that your Higher Self can see farther and knows more than your ego personality.

Freedom also involves transcending your survival issues. The mechanism used by your ego to grab your attention is fear, which energetically constricts and binds you. Fear pulls inward rather than allowing for expansion. And the more you fear, the more you imprison yourself.

Love, however, is the expression of your freedom. The more deeply you can feel and passionately express love, the freer your life will be. Love creates the space for laughter so you can see humor in your mistakes.

Universal Freedom lies in a subtle but awesome shift of perception from seeing and feeling yourself as separate from Source, to knowing that you are unified with every aspect of Source. In this unity with the Source of your Being, you reunite those fragments of self you have denied.

In feeling the love of the universe and the unfolding flow of the Great Plan, you begin to fully express your infinite freedom. And, to the extent that you can free yourself of self imposed bondage, you will be able to help others move beyond their walls of self-imprisonment.

Card for the Day

If you chose this card you may be feeling restricted in some part of your life, as if you have lost your freedom. Perhaps you feel victimized by circumstances you perceive are beyond your control. Victim and victimizer roles stem from early childhood experiences and, although they appear powerfully real, they are still dramas in which you have cast yourself through choice.

Your Divine Self guided you to this symbol card, silently suggesting it is time to step out of the soap opera and into your freedom. It is important to obtain clarity as to your judgments, fears, and beliefs, which are creating the walls of your own prison. Become aware of them, acknowledge them, forgive them and release them.

Meditation

Find a quiet spot and study the symbol. Hold the symbol up to your heart (symbol facing your body) and ask your Divine Self, *"Beloved Divine Self, I now choose to fully express my freedom for my highest good. I ask that the purest and clearest frequencies of this symbol be transferred through all levels of my Being. I choose to be shown my fears and illusions so I can move through them with grace and ease. So be it. And so it is."*

Allow yourself to be open to receive direction from the Source of your Being.

Color and Symbol Balancing

Yellow is the primary color of this symbol. Issues about being free and claiming personal spiritual power are often held in the solar plexus. Yellow helps open the solar plexus to allow for the release of emotional complexes.

The symbol's secondary color is salmon pink, which activates the sexual chakra, one of the important centers of creativity in the body.

Red, the tertiary color, assists in opening the root chakra and grounding you to the Earth.

It is recommended, when projecting this symbol's frequency,

to see it carried on a current of bright yellow light. Visualize the yellow light filling the solar plexus area like a miniature sun, radiating out through the body. Imagine yellow light carrying the symbol's vibration and radiating the symbol's frequency out through the whole auric field.

Yellow can help clarify the mental body and assist in the release of mental polarities. Silently intend, as you project the symbol, that the recipient of the symbol's energy align with his/her highest good and greatest freedom.

Use the colors salmon pink and red only if it appears that the root (red) or sexual (salmon pink) chakras are energetically blocked and need to be cleared.

CARD #13
I Am Aligned with the Christos

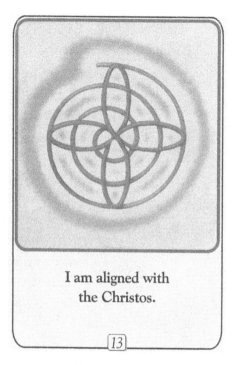

I am aligned with
the Christos.

13

AFFIRMATION

"I accept and embody my true Christos nature."

Insight

This symbol is attuned to the Universal Christos frequency, which was integrated into the Earth's energy field by Jesus. The Universal Christos Essence is expressed through many spiritual and matter dimensions, and exists throughout all space and time.

Although we each embody the Christos frequency at our Core, limiting cultural beliefs which we have accepted govern our perception of reality and restrict us from manifesting this, our True Nature. As we clear our illusions of powerlessness, abandon-

CORRESPONDENCES

PRIMARY COLOR	Gold
SECONDARY COLOR	Purple
TERTIARY COLOR	Red
METALS\CRYSTALS USED IN GRIDS:	Gold (metal)
	Golden Barite
	Golden Topaz
	Golden Lithium Crystal
CHAKRAS CLEARED AND ALIGNED:	Crown Chakra
	Heart Chakra
	Root Chakra
MERIDIANS CLEARED AND ALIGNED:	Stomach Meridian
	Spleen Meridian
	Heart Meridian
	Kidney Meridian
	Pericardium Meridian
	Triple Warmer Meridian
PRIMARY ELEMENTS REPRESENTED BY THE SYMBOL:	Fire/Air/Water/Earth

ment, and sense of limitation, our eternal Core Christos Nature can shine through and manifest.

Many religions speak of the tri-fold nature of Source. Each in their own language speak of the One, the Monad, the Source, reflecting itself in three aspects: Divine Father, Divine Mother, and Divine Child. Some schools of metaphysics speak of these three aspects as the three rays or the three-fold flame.

The Divine Child, or the Universal Christos aspect, represents the balanced expression of the Divine Father and Divine Mother aspects. The Divine Father and Divine Mother polarities are resolved in unity within the Divine Child, the Universal Christos.

Jesus, through the purification of his thoughts, emotions and physical body, was able to become a clear vessel for the Christos frequency and awareness, and in turn demonstrated what we each are potentially capable of becoming. His resurrection proved that the paradigm of physical death can be transcended. He demonstrated the multi-dimensional nature of the Christos, with his ability to bridge and move between dimensions.

It is through an open and loving heart that your Christos nature can more easily manifest. The most powerful and overriding quality of the life of Jesus was his ability to love. He loved those who shunned him and those who welcomed him, both his enemies and his friends. Through his love, he merged all polarities in his life and in the universe.

Jesus, as a way-shower, demonstrated what is possible when you allow your Christos Nature to become the dominant force in your life. However, it is impossible to manifest your Christos Nature if you remain in judgment, anger, or fear.

This *Waveform Symbol* embodies the intention to align fully with the Christos at the Core of Your Being: to be true to yourself, and to resurrect yourself out of the paradigm of isolation, death, and entropy into the paradigm of love, unity, and eternal life.

The symbol expresses the choice to align with your Christos Nature as the uppermost goal of your life, and to make all other goals secondary. It also includes the intention to love the Source of your Being, others, and yourself, with all your heart and soul, thereby unifying the polarities in your life. It represents both the beginning and the end of the path, the alpha and omega of your Being.

Card for the Day

If your Divine Self guided you to this symbol, it is a gentle suggestion from your soul to re-order your priorities and realign with your Christos Nature. Our culture has a multitude of belief systems on how you should live your life, what to strive for, how to be unique and different, and how to rise above the masses. A close evaluation of these beliefs will prove that they are based upon fear, separation, and one-up-manship.

The way of the world is not necessarily the way of Spirit. Your Divine Self, your Christos Nature, knows that all people and all life are extensions of Source. There is no separation. Love is the unifying force of the universe. Spirit is continually redirecting you back to the truth that you are one with all things, and through that unity all things are possible. The selection of this symbol card is such a reminder.

Meditation

Study the symbol, its form and its color. Attune to its energy. Bring the symbol card to your heart (symbol facing your body) and ask your soul, *"Beloved Divine Self, I choose to embody the purest, clearest, and highest essence of this symbol to align with my Christos Nature and manifest it in my life. I choose now to clear all beliefs and emotions in resistance to the full embodiment of the Christos. So be it. And so it is!"*

Visualize the gold color of the symbol and the symbol's energy entering your heart and flowing through your body. Allow the gold light to transmute and clear any blocks within your body. Feel the Christos Nature at the Core of Your Being radiate out and fill your life.

Color and Symbol Balancing

Gold, the symbol's primary color, resonates with the Gold Ray of Christ Consciousness. It assists in the merging of polarities and in the healing of fractures within your Being.

Purple, the symbol's secondary color, allows for profound cleansing and purification. It assists in aligning you to your soul's mission and Divine Essence.

Red, the symbol's tertiary color, activates and opens the root chakra, helping you ground the pure Christos Energy into the Earth plane and into your daily life.

It is recommended that you work primarily with the Gold and Purple Rays when broadcasting the vibration of this symbol.

Begin with red only if the individual appears very ungrounded or un-centered. Should this be the case, project the symbol on the Red Ray. Direct the Red Ray into the root chakra, allowing the root chakra to expand. Then visualize a cord of red light running from the root chakra into the center of the Earth, anchoring the person solidly into the Earth's core.

If grounding is not required, begin by directing the symbol's vibration on a current of purple light. Visualize the purple light infusing the whole body, including every cell (down to the DNA level). Hold the intention that the Purple Ray melt and dissolve every blockage resisting the embodiment of the Christos. Accept and feel this happening.

After the purification with the Purple Ray feels complete, broadcast the symbol's frequency via the Gold Christ Ray. Allow the Gold Ray to enter at the heart and then expand and radiate out through the whole body. Finish by visualizing the individual as a radiant gold Being, transmitting gold light into the deepest reaches of the universe.

CARD #14

I Channel the Energies of Spirit into Form

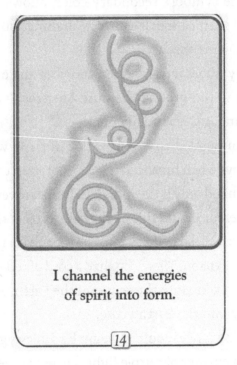

I channel the energies
of spirit into form.

14

AFFIRMATION

*"I choose to remain open on all levels to allow the Light
of Spirit to flow into and manifest in my physical form."*

Insight

This symbol assists in opening the major chakras, increasing the amount of spiritual energy (chi, ki) flowing through you and into the Earth. The essence of the symbol is about accepting your body as spiritualized matter and choosing to ground yourself fully in the physical. It is about being "okay" with your physical form and allowing the Light of Spirit (life force) to flow easily through you. Emotionally, the maximal flow of spiritual

CORRESPONDENCES

PRIMARY COLOR	Gold
SECONDARY COLOR	Magenta
TERTIARY COLOR	Violet
METALS\CRYSTALS USED IN GRIDS:	Gold (metal)
	Golden Beryl
	Golden Topaz
	Gold Rutilated Quartz
	Yellow Tiger's Eye
CHAKRAS CLEARED AND ALIGNED:	Crown Chakra
	Solar Plexus Chakra
MERIDIANS CLEARED AND ALIGNED:	Kidney Meridian
	Pericardium Meridian
	Liver Meridian
PRIMARY ELEMENTS REPRESENTED BY THE SYMBOL:	Ether/Fire/Water

energy through your being comes through allowing and accepting without resistance.

The Light activating property of the symbol helps to free you from the illusion that you are at the mercy of matter. There are many mass consciousness beliefs concerning our bondage to the physical. If you choose to believe you are constrained by the physical, you will experience those constraints in your life.

The use of this symbol will help unlock the knowing that your consciousness, arising from Source, can influence the molecules of your Being. You are not really limited by the properties of matter. The miracles of the Masters, such as the transmutation of water to wine, prove that consciousness can directly influence the physicality of form.

When you shift your level of consciousness, the physical body will also shift. The symbol helps to clear, on the DNA level, family/racial memories and beliefs that you are controlled by your genetic lineage. As limiting beliefs are cleared, so too, are the blockages to the flow of life force.

The amplification and increase of the flow of spiritual energy through your body promotes rejuvenation and regeneration. The increased flow of Light also enhances your ability to manifest your desires. When you carry more Light, it becomes easier to energize your dreams and manifest your visions.

This symbol embodies the intention to remain open at all levels, within all chakras, and energy bodies. It embodies the choice to absorb and channel spiritual Light within and through your cells, tissues, and form.

Card for the Day

If your Divine Self guided you to select this card, it is time to let go of fear on all levels and to ground and anchor God's Light fully into your physical form. Visualize your physical body as compressed Light, as bright as any star. Acknowledge that you made the choice to work and play in a physical form. Know that as you allow the Light of Source to flow easily through you, you are helping to anchor the vibration of Heaven on Earth.

Meditation

Sit quietly, hold the symbol card to your heart (symbol facing your body) and affirm the following, "*Beloved Divine Self, I now choose to open fully to the flow of Spirit. I allow the Light of Spirit to flow through me and to be grounded into my physical form. So be it. And so it is.*"

Feel the energy of the symbol resonate through your whole

body. Allow your root chakra, at the base of your spine, to open. Experience your connection to Earth. See your crown chakra open and draw in the gold Christ Light. Visualize gold light flowing through you, from your crown, down your spine, out the root, and into the Earth.

When you first begin this meditation, you may have old fears (blockages in energy flow) such as feeling unworthy or not good enough, come up to be addressed. Choose to ground the fear and anxiety out of your body. See these old energies being easily carried by the current of gold light into the Earth. Acknowledge that these fears and beliefs no longer serve you, and that it is time to let them go.

Color and Symbol Balancing

Gold is the primary color of the symbol. It helps you align strongly with the Christ energy, the Great Central Sun, and the Core of Your Being.

Magenta, the symbol's secondary color, results from the combination of violet and red. The violet aspect of the Magenta Ray helps to open the crown chakra; the red aspect assists in expanding the root, or base chakra. Thus, magenta activates the central energy core of the body along the spine.

The tertiary color of the symbol is violet, for clearing and transmutation of blockages.

When projecting the symbol, it is recommended that the vibration of the symbol first be transmitted on the Violet Ray. Visualize any constrictions in the flow of energy along the spine dissolving and melting away. Then, intend that the symbol's frequency be carried on the Magenta Ray. See the magenta color opening the crown and root (base) chakras as the Magenta Ray fills the spine.

As a last step, project the symbol's essence on a current of gold light. Sense the gold light flowing into the crown, down the spine, out the root, and into the Earth. Visualize the Gold Christ Ray expanding out through the body to the edges of space.

CARD #15

The Perfection in My Core Essence Is Reflected in My Perfect Body

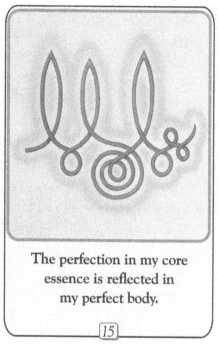

The perfection in my core
essence is reflected in
my perfect body.

15

AFFIRMATION

"I now accept, on all levels of my being, that I am Divine. I allow my physical body to be a full expression of my Divinity."

Insight

This symbol carries the frequency of accepting and embodying one's divinity in the physical. It expresses the intention of having all of your energy bodies[3] in alignment, one with each other and with the Source of your Being.

One model of consciousness is that your divine true essence

---

3 *Spiritual, mental, emotional, etheric and physical.*

CORRESPONDENCES

PRIMARY COLOR	Emerald Green
SECONDARY COLOR	Gold
TERTIARY COLOR	Light Magenta
METALS\CRYSTALS USED IN GRIDS:	Green Tourmaline
	Green Jade
	Dioptase
	Peridot
	Emerald
	Gold (metal)
CHAKRAS CLEARED AND ALIGNED:	Crown Chakra
	Heart Chakra
MERIDIANS CLEARED AND ALIGNED:	Heart Meridian
	Triple Warmer Meridian
PRIMARY ELEMENTS REPRESENTED	
BY THE SYMBOL:	Ether/Fire

exists at the Core of Your Being. Wrapped around this sacred core are the beliefs and illusions of separation and limitation you have accepted since childhood. The world is viewed through these distorted wrappings. For example, you may feel separate from your divinity, you believe you need to age, or you may see yourself as unworthy of love. By focusing on these beliefs, you energize and manifest them.

The beliefs of mass consciousness suggest that your bodies are not sacred. This symbol carries the reverse message and truth: that your body is spiritually clean and perfect and is the vessel for Source, as divine as any other aspect of heaven. Focusing on and energizing these truths allows them to manifest into form.

Accepting and loving your body as divine, holy, and sacred initiates some important shifts. You will find yourself accepting and allowing Earth energy into your Being and becoming more strongly grounded to Mother Earth. You will also begin integrating the masculine and feminine energies more fully, accepting their balance into your inner and outer life. You will probably find it easier to relate to the opposite sex.

Supporting the belief that your body is divine will result in the clearing of the congested and blocked energy within your body. A stronger and more powerful life force will begin to flow through your physical being, giving your body a chance to regenerate and rejuvenate. In time, your physical body can become healthier and stronger, potentially free from physical ailments.

Loving your physical form as a vessel of Source allows you to clear self-judgments and enjoy your body more. In this state of expansion, your soul essence and physical body will feel aligned. You will find yourself more creative because you are welcoming a more solid connection with Earth. It will be easier for you to manifest your heart's desires.

The essence of this symbol acknowledges that your sacred, holy, and Divine Nature has now manifested fully in your physical form. It is truly knowing that your body is the holy vessel that carries the infinite spirit of Source. It is embracing the truth that all dimensions have merged into one, and that God is no longer outside of you.

Card for the Day

If you pulled this card, you are ready to accept yourself as a holy expression of the great and infinite Spirit in physical form. It is an excellent time to stand before a full length mirror and say, "*The perfection of my soul essence is manifesting as my perfect body.*" See the radiance of Spirit shining through you and acknowledge that heaven lies within. See yourself as a divine and perfect vessel. Accept and love your physical form. Your body is a miracle. It is the manifestation of Light as matter, and the unification of dimensions.

Make the intention to honor your body every day. Affirm: "*I am spiritually clear and perfect on every level.*" Feel this affirmation soak into every cell, down to the DNA level. As you walk through the day, sense the perfection that pulsates through your form.

Meditation

Find a quiet place and time in your life to study the shape and color of the symbol. Hold the symbol to your heart (symbol facing your body), and affirm to yourself, "*Beloved Divine Self, I now choose to acknowledge the divinity that is expressed through my body. I now allow the essence of my flawless spirit to fill my Being and to transform my body into its divine and perfected form. So be it. And so it is.*"

Visualize, as you inhale, the emerald green color of the symbol flowing into your heart and through your whole body. Choose to be filled as well with the quality and essence of the symbol. See, in your mind's eye, your body shifting and transforming into the perfected shape and form you choose to manifest. Allow the divine blueprint of your perfected being to sink deep into your cells and tissues. Feel and know yourself expressing your divine, sacred, and perfected form.

Color and Symbol Balancing

Emerald green is the primary color of the symbol. It helps to balance and harmonize the body. It works on the heart chakra as well, opening it, bringing sky and Earth energies into equilibrium.

The secondary color of the symbol is the Gold Christ Ray, the spiritual color of the soul.

Magenta, the symbol's tertiary color, is created through the merging of red (which opens the root chakra to the Earth energy) and violet (which opens the crown chakra to the sky energy). Magenta thus activates the sky and Earth currents that run up and down the spine.

A powerful clearing process involves first projecting the symbol's vibration on a current of magenta light, seeing the light fill the spine, opening the crown and root chakras. Follow the color of magenta by projecting the symbol on a ray of gold light, infusing the whole body with gold.

Lastly, project the symbol's vibration on a stream of emerald green light, visualizing it filling the heart and then flooding the entire body, all organs, glands, tissues, and cells. Set the intention that the body is in perfect balance and harmony while you project the frequency of the symbol.

CARD #16
I Resolve All Inner Conflict to Peace.

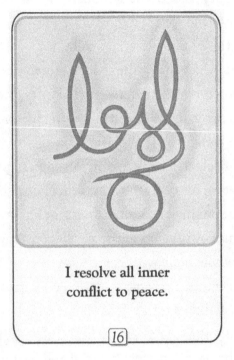

I resolve all inner
conflict to peace.

16

AFFIRMATION

"I turn my conflicts over to my Divine Self to be resolved."

Insight

The essence of this card assists you in coming from your heart where there is no fear, and letting go of all disagreement, struggle, and opposition. Your disagreements with others arise from the playing field of the mind. When you move to your heart, you perceive the world differently. It becomes easier to let go and let God handle the details.

Krishnamurti once said, "War is waged in the world because

CORRESPONDENCES

PRIMARY COLOR	Pink
SECONDARY COLOR	Lemon Yellow
TERTIARY COLOR	Blue
METALS\CRYSTALS USED IN GRIDS:	Rose Quartz
	Rhodochrosite
	Pink Tourmaline
	Pink Kunzite
CHAKRAS CLEARED AND ALIGNED:	Heart Chakra
	Solar Plexus Chakra
MERIDIANS CLEARED AND ALIGNED:	Lung Meridian
	Large Intestine Meridian
	Heart Meridian
	Gall Bladder Meridian
	Liver Meridian
PRIMARY ELEMENTS REPRESENTED BY THE SYMBOL:	Fire/Water

war is waged in men's minds."

All conflict could be said to be first internal, only later becoming externalized. It arises because you feel separate from others and perceive differences in ideas and beliefs. This engenders fear and mistrust.

This symbol enhances the ability to get out of the way and to focus on similarities rather than on differences. It assists in centering in the heart, and in trusting the universe. It helps you see beneath the surface to the inter-connectedness of all things.

The symbol is specifically designed to help resolve conflicted feelings in your relationships by moving the point of awareness from the mind to the heart.

When you feel hurt, fearful, or angry at another, you project your separation outward upon them. Usually the other person, sensing that projection, reacts to it and projects it back. And so the drama that is out-pictured results from a fractured perception of the world.

This symbol expands and warms the heart. The spiritual heart is grounded in love and unity, and can thus heal the conflict that has been created. Through a peaceful heart, you can forgive and let go of the judgments you have overlaid on others as you surrender to the Source of your Being.

Card for the Day

If you chose this symbol, you are close to healing an inner conflict with yourself, with another, or with some aspect of your life (your job, your living situation). Take heart! Know the conflict can be resolved. Focus on your heart and choose to love and honor yourself. Choose to forgive yourself and everyone in your life.

Meditation

Hold the symbol card up to your heart (symbol facing your body) and ask your Divine Self the following, "*Beloved Divine Self, assist me in clearing and resolving to love the conflict I feel. Transfer the purest and clearest frequencies of this symbol to all levels of my Being. I choose to fully embody the deepest level of peace in my heart. So be it. And so it is!*"

Sit in meditation and allow the energy of the symbol to flow through your whole body. When you feel yourself become calm, ask your soul, your Divine Self, for an answer to your situation.

Realize that as you find the peace within, the conflict in your outer life will dissipate. Know that your Divine Self has the answer. Choose to enter a deeper level of peace in your life. Let go, and let the solution appear.

Color and Symbol Balancing

The primary color of this symbol is pink. The color pink soothes and calms the heart and opens it to love and acceptance. Pink works on the emotional level of the heart, helping to heal wounds and feelings of separation.

The symbol's secondary color is lemon, which helps purge and purify the solar plexus chakra where most judgment is held.

And the symbol's tertiary color is sky blue, which helps to clear blocks in the throat chakra to expressing one's truth.

When projecting the symbol's frequency, visualize it first on a current of pink light which fills the heart area.

After it feels like the heart has expanded, move your focus to the solar plexus chakra, projecting the symbol on a Ray of Lemon Light. And if it appears that the throat is blocked, then infuse the throat chakra with a sky blue color as well as the vibration of the symbol.

Complete the color balancing by returning to the Pink Ray, filling the body and aura with rich pink light.

CARD #17

I Align All Levels of My Being with Source

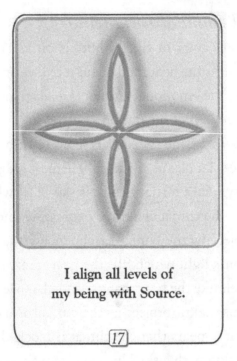

I align all levels of
my being with Source.

17

AFFIRMATION

"I align my physical, emotional, mental, and spiritual levels, one with each other, and with the Source of my Being."

Insight

The energetic quality of this symbol assists you in bringing your four basic energy bodies (physical, emotional, mental, and spiritual) into alignment with each other and with the Christos energy.[4] If you feel alone, isolated, unloved, or fearful, then there has been a misalignment of your energy bodies. When you bring

---

4   *See Chapter 3 for a description of the energy bodies*

CORRESPONDENCES

PRIMARY COLOR	Gold
SECONDARY COLOR	Purple
TERTIARY COLOR	Silver
METALS\CRYSTALS USED IN GRIDS:	Gold & Silver (metal)
	Gold Mica
	Golden Barite
	Peach Calcite
CHAKRAS CLEARED AND ALIGNED:	Crown Chakra
	Heart Chakra
MERIDIANS CLEARED AND ALIGNED:	Lung Meridian
	Spleen Meridian
	Heart Meridian
	Kidney Meridian
	Pericardium Meridian
PRIMARY ELEMENTS REPRESENTED BY THE SYMBOL:	Air/Fire/Water/Earth

your energy bodies into alignment, there arises a sense of unity. This feeling of At-One-Ment is a feeling of being in your center.

Energy on the higher dimensional levels is transferred through resonance. To fully access the power, love and wisdom of the universe (the Divine Trinity), you must first come into resonance with the Universal Field so the transfer can occur. This symbol assists in this alignment.

You can consciously feel your divinity and a sense of wholeness when you feel energetically aligned with the universe. The emotional states of fear, anger, and isolation result from feeling disconnected and out-of-alignment with the Source of your Being and the Universal Field.

This symbol embodies alignment with the Universal Field

through the four Universal states. The four Universal states are often expressed as the four cardinal directions (North, South, East, West) and have been recognized in spiritual literature since the time of Buddha, approximately 4,000 years ago.

They have been ascribed with qualities associated with energy transition states: Earth (solid), water (liquid), air (gas), and fire (kinetic). They have also been equated with angelic energies: Archangel Michael, Archangel Gabriel, Archangel Raphael, and Archangel Uriel. A symbol often used to depict the four Universal states is an equal armed cross within a circle.

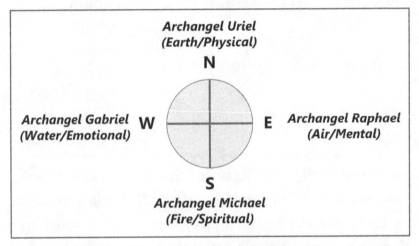

The diagram above represents the four Universal states in perfect balance and harmony. When the four Universal states are in balance, so too, are the electrical and magnetic, the cosmic and Earth, and the masculine and feminine energies. The various vibrational levels within your Being (physical, emotional, mental, and spiritual) can also be associated with these four Universal states. So to be in alignment on all levels of your Being is to also be in alignment with the four Universal states.

When you come into vibrational harmony and balance on all levels with the Source of your being, the life force energy can flow freely through your physical body. This enhances regeneration and rejuvenation and can slow down the aging process.

This is the symbol of divine integration, wholeness and perfect balance. It represents the fluid movement and union of the four Universal states. It is the symbol of the Holy Spirit manifested into form.

Card for the Day

If this card has surfaced today, you may be experiencing a sense of discord and non-alignment with the Universal Flow. Know that through intention, you can achieve harmony, a sense of "groundedness" and well being. The following meditation is recommended.

Meditation

Look carefully at the symbol. The symbol's center represents the nexus and balancing point of the four Universal states of the cosmic and Earth energies.

Imagine yourself in the center of the symbol. See a large expanded version of the symbol surrounding you as you sit. Feel yourself in the symbol's center and allow the energy of the symbol to course through you. Connect with your soul essence through your heart and make the following request: "*Beloved Divine Self, I now choose to align all levels of my Being with Divine Will. I choose that this occur now. So be it. And so it is!*"

Allow your heart chakra to open like a flower and absorb the gold Christ Light associated with this symbol. Choose to be at one with All-That-Is. Feel a sense of unity with the Universal Field.

Color and Symbol Balancing

The primary color of this symbol is the Gold Christ Ray, which can assist you in being in balance and harmony with your Divine Self and soul purpose.

Purple is the symbol's secondary color; it helps you experience your divinity.

Silver, the symbol's tertiary color, represents the Divine Feminine essence.

Before projecting the symbol to its recipient, silently make the intention that the individual's energy bodies (physical, etheric, emotional, mental, and spiritual) come into alignment with each other and with Divine Will. Visualize the symbol's vibration being carried on a current of gold light. See the gold light infuse the individual's spine.

Next, visualize the gold light extending up from their crown to the Great Central Sun, and extending down from their root chakra into the Earth's Core. See the individual fully aligned in a column of gold light running from the Great Central Sun to the Earth's Core. Hold this visualization until it feels as if it has "set into place." (See *The Sacred Core Visualization*, pages 45-46.)

If the individual feels upset or fearful in the beginning of the session, you may want to begin with purple light to help purge the discord. Imagine the symbol's vibration carried on a waterfall of purple light that cascades down, over and through the person, flushing out all conflict and fear.

When the old emotional energies have been cleared, then follow with the gold light visualization.

CARD #18

I Give Unconditionally for I Am Totally Supported by the Universe

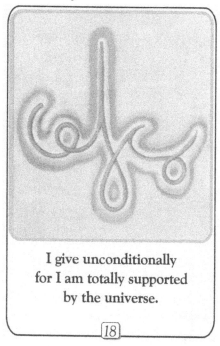

I give unconditionally
for I am totally supported
by the universe.

18

AFFIRMATION

"I trust completely in the Universe and Source in meeting my needs and I am able to remain open to giving and receiving on all levels."

Insight

The essence of this card is about opening up and trusting the universe to support you on every level. When you trust deeply that you are supported by Source, then no sense of fear, lack, or loss exists. You realize you can give unconditionally without losing.

Love implies an equal and opposite exchange of energy in harmony and balance between the lover and the beloved. You

CORRESPONDENCES	
PRIMARY COLOR	Green
SECONDARY COLOR	Violet
TERTIARY COLOR	Yellow-Gold
METALS\CRYSTALS USED IN GRIDS:	Emerald
	Turquoise
	Green Jade
	Larimar
	Aquamarine
CHAKRAS CLEARED AND ALIGNED:	Heart Chakra
	Throat Chakra
MERIDIANS CLEARED AND ALIGNED:	Large Intestine Meridian
	Heart Meridian
	Kidney Meridian
	Triple Warmer Meridian
PRIMARY ELEMENTS REPRESENTED BY THE SYMBOL:	Air/Fire/Water

give at the same level as you receive; you receive to the same degree that you give. When this occurs, the bonding is absolute. Indeed, the universe is held together by love.

This flow, however, can be blocked in three basic ways:

1. You are willing to receive, but have difficulty giving.
2. You give easily but have trouble receiving.
3. You block both your receiving and giving.

All of these blockages in flow occur because of beliefs and fears of separation, e.g., feeling separate from God, from others, and from self. Past traumas leave you feeling "burned," and defensive shields are created to keep the past from reoccurring. Paradoxically, these "shields" and "defenses" block the energy flow, the love, and manifest the very circumstances which are feared.

When you trust the universe and the Source of your Being completely, you experience being part of the Universal Flow. There is no resistance. The flow is effortless and automatic. Everything seems to click into place. You have an inner sense of what to do and, as you do it, you are fully assisted. You feel connected to the flow, and to Infinite Power. You expand beyond the small self and sense the greater design, the infinite current, which is the foundation that is supporting all things.

The illusion of scarcity is predicated on the belief that love, money, and energy are limited in supply, that they will run out. For example, you may believe that if your friend loves someone else, there won't be enough left over for you. Energy, love and wisdom are infinite in universal supply. However, the universe also supports you by manifesting whatever you believe. If you choose to believe in scarcity, the universe will create exactly the scarcity that you fear.

You can move into an open flow with the universe by trusting that you will receive what you need and knowing you can give unconditionally without fear of loss. Know that the more you love, the more love will be mirrored back to you; the more you give, the more you will receive. Be open and grateful for the abundance in your life. Allow the abundance of universal supply to flow to you and it will.

Card for the Day

If you have chosen this card, it is time to jump into the flow of universal supply and allow the current to support you. Instead of frantically splashing in fear of drowning, relax and lie back. Allow yourself to float. Know it is safe to love and be loved. Acknowledge that you are worthy of receiving the abundance of the universe simply because you are a child of God. Your worthiness to receive doesn't depend on what you have done or what you have learned in school. You have always been worthy of receiving the infinite supply of the universe, simply because you exist. Trust that the immeasurable love of Source is ever-present. Know it is safe to give from your heart, for that love will be returned many fold. Trust that nothing is risked when you give.

Meditation

The following visualization is founded upon the truth that God is the Source of your supply. The Source of your supply is not your job, your boss, or your stocks. Nor is it the number of widgets you sell. Energy flows from God, through your life, back to God. One of the many expressions of that energy flow happens to be money.

Study the color and shape of the symbol. In a quiet place, bring the symbol up to your heart, with the symbol facing your body. State silently to yourself, *"I now choose to embody the highest and purest essence of this symbol. I acknowledge that my abundance comes from Source and flows through me and others back to Source. I affirm I am always supported by Source whether I receive or give. So be it. And so it is."*

Visualize the emerald green color from this symbol filling your body and life. You can also visualize money flowing from Source through a company, job or business to you and through your life.

Likewise, see yourself paying the bills, allowing the money to go to a person or company and then flowing back to Source. See a grand loop of money cycling around and around, from God, through your life, and back to God. Feel your support from the universe. Know that as you give, you will receive.

Color and Symbol Balancing

The primary color of this symbol is emerald green. Emerald green expands the heart chakra and helps to activate self-love. Self-love, in turn, creates the space of openness to give and receive without fear.

The secondary color for this symbol is violet, a color that can effectively transmute blocked or stuck energy.

The symbol's tertiary color, yellow-gold, helps to open the solar plexus chakra and release fears held there.

If blocks are perceived in the chakras or body, you may want to begin projecting the symbol on a current of violet light. Visualize the violet light entering the blocked areas, breaking them up in intense explosions, and transmuting them into light.

If the solar plexus appears to hold emotional complexes such as "fear," "anger," or "neediness," you can use the Yellow-Gold Ray to open and expand this chakra. This will assist in the release of these issues. Alternating between yellow-gold and violet light will help bring up and clear solar plexus blocks.

The last and most important color to use with the symbol is its primary color, green. See and feel the symbol's vibration on a current of green light. Imagine the green light expanding out from the heart chakra, enveloping all the chakras and unifying them. Feel the essence of the universe's infinite abundance carried within the Green Ray, filling the individual's entire body and being.

CARD #19

I Am Aligned with My Divine Core Essence

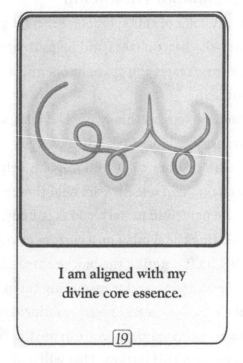

I am aligned with my
divine core essence.

19

AFFIRMATION

"I align with the Divine, Sacred, and Holy Essence at the Core of my Being."

Insight

This symbol acknowledges the truth that your Core Essence is an extension of Source. Your Core Being is divine, sacred, and holy. The symbol further embodies the intention of accepting and fully aligning with the highest expression of your Core.

Choosing to accept the truth that your Core is connected to the highest Source and to align with this truth is the fundamental step to manifesting it fully in your life. All the saints,

CORRESPONDENCES

PRIMARY COLOR	Rose Pink
SECONDARY COLOR	Yellow-Gold
TERTIARY COLOR	Indigo
METALS\CRYSTALS USED IN GRIDS:	Rose Quartz
	Pink Coral
	Watermelon Tourmaline
	Pink Kunzite
	Rhodochrosite
CHAKRAS CLEARED AND ALIGNED:	Root Chakra
	Heart Chakra
	Brow Chakra
MERIDIANS CLEARED AND ALIGNED:	Heart Meridian
	Small Intestine Meridian
	Pericardium Meridian
	Liver Meridian
PRIMARY ELEMENTS REPRESENTED BY THE SYMBOL:	Air/Fire

holy women and men, have recognized their divinity and thus manifested this reality in their life.

The life you experience is a result of the seed thoughts and beliefs you have planted. The flower that blooms and the fruit that ripens is an "out-picturing" of the seed. If you feel separate from Source and plant this belief in your subconscious, this seed can only bear the barren fruit of feeling unsupported by the universe. However, if you accept the truth that you are an extension of Source, this seed will ripen into a life that feels whole and complete. You will attain a knowing that "I and my Father are one."

This symbol activates and energizes the core energy circuit in your physical being, which runs up and down your spine in a two-way energy flow. (Earth energy flows up the spine—root to crown. The sky energy flows down the spine—crown to root.)

The vibrational quality of the symbol expands the core energy circuit, opening both the major and minor chakras. The increased life force resulting from this energy flow supports a strong bond to the Earth and the cosmos, leading to a deep sense of peace.

Card for the Day

If you selected this card, your Divine Self is guiding you to realign with your Divine Core Essence, which is an extension and expression of Source. When you acknowledge that the foundation of your Being is Source and choose to align with it, you open yourself to infinite possibilities and the potential for miracles.

The choice to accept your divinity sets powerful forces into motion and brings your whole life into alignment with your True Nature.

Meditation

In a quiet location, study the color and form of the symbol. When you feel ready, bring the card up to your heart with the symbol facing your body. Relax and breathe slowly. As you inhale, see and feel the symbol's vibration enter your heart on a ray of rose-pink light. Allow your heart to expand as it fills with the light and essence of the symbol.

Say to yourself, "*I choose to sink into the stillness at the center of my Being.*" ... Pause ... allow your self to feel the Christ essence ... and continue, "*I now align my life expression with my Divine Core Essence. So be it. And so it is.*"

Visualize the rose-pink light becoming yellow-gold in color. Then see a column of yellow-gold light running up and down your spine. Imagine the upper portion of the column extending up to the Central Sun at the center of the universe.

Visualize the lower portion of the column extending down from your tailbone to the center of the Earth. (See *The Sacred Core Visualization*, page 45-46.)

Rest in the stillness of your Divine Core and feel your Divine Core Essence connected through all time and space to the Earth and the cosmos.

Color and Symbol Balancing

Rose pink is the primary color of this symbol. The reddish tone of the color helps to open the root chakra, deepening your connection to the Earth. The pink quality of the color activates and opens the heart chakra, particularly on the emotional level.

Yellow-gold is the secondary color of the symbol. The yellowish tone helps to clear and expand the solar plexus chakra. The gold color activates all the chakras with an emphasis on the heart and the chakras above the head.

Indigo is the tertiary color for the symbol and helps to clear and energize the brow, or the third eye, chakra.

It is recommended that you first project the vibration of the symbol on a Rose-Pink Ray of light. Visualize the Rose-Pink Ray (with the symbol's essence) infusing the root and heart chakras, allowing these chakras to open. Follow with the Yellow-Gold Ray.

Project the symbol's vibration on a current of yellow-gold light, filling the solar plexus chakra and then the whole energetic core of the individual with light. Expand the light out from the spine so it infuses and fills the whole body.

CARD #20
I Now See Clearly

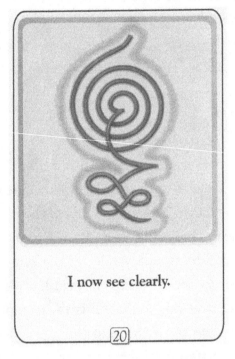

I now see clearly.

20

AFFIRMATION

"I go within and draw upon my intuitive knowing to see the big picture."

Insight

The essence of this symbol assists you in opening to the intuition and guidance of your soul to obtain clarity about any life situation. The symbol's frequency assists in clearing fears and confusion when faced with a challenging circumstance. When the fear is cleared, clarity rises effortlessly into your consciousness.

It is a natural state of grace to see through the eyes of your soul. Infinite knowing is ever-present; only doubts and fears

CORRESPONDENCES

PRIMARY COLOR	Indigo
SECONDARY COLOR	Purple
TERTIARY COLOR	Light Lemon
METALS\CRYSTALS USED IN GRIDS:	Sugilite-Luvulite
	Sodalite
	Lapis Lazuli
	Azurite
CHAKRAS CLEARED AND ALIGNED:	Brow Chakra
	Throat Chakra
MERIDIANS CLEARED AND ALIGNED:	Triple Warmer Meridian
PRIMARY ELEMENTS REPRESENTED	
BY THE SYMBOL:	Ether/Air/Fire

block clear perception. As these doubts and fears dissolve, your field of vision expands, your insight improves, and you can see from the perspective of your Greater Self rather than only from the limited perceptions of your smaller self.

If you come from the false belief that you are small, insignificant and powerless, you will be drawn to the conclusion that someone or some thing outside of you holds the answers. By going within and drawing on the Source of your Being for guidance, you will discover you don't have to rely on the small self for answers, nor do you have to rely on others for guidance. You hold the clarity of vision that you seek.

The energy of this symbol also helps you to stand back and see the Big Picture, to see how all the facets of any situation are connected.

Imagine a camera focused on a thorn bush. All that can be seen are its leaves and twisted branches. As the focus is drawn back, there is a panoramic view which includes mountains, sky, valley, trees, and grass. The thorn bush is now seen within the context of a larger field.

Likewise, when you continuously focus on a problem, it begins to fill your entire viewing screen, looming out of proportion and becoming overwhelming. However, as you draw back, the issue diminishes and you can begin to see it in relationship to the total field.

The issue which looms so large from one perspective can shrink to insignificant proportion with a shift of focus (or attention). When your field of vision is large enough you can see how to circumvent the problem—how to walk around the thorn bush.

Seeing the Big Picture can also involve becoming aware of the cycles and rhythms of change. You often unconsciously fall into patterns that have a long cycle (e.g., occurring every three years), patterns you are not conscious of because of their infrequency, or you create a behavioral dance with another that is repeated over and over again. When you are emotionally immersed in the dance, you don't see its recurring cycle. However, when you step back, you can become aware of the pattern and can then choose to continue to dance—or not.

The *"I Now See Clearly"* symbol is about relying on your soul's insight and deep inner knowing. It's realizing that standing on the top of the mountain, the perspective provided by your Divine Self, allows you to see further than standing in a box canyon.

Card for the Day

If you chose this card, there may be an issue or situation in your life that, when viewed from a broader perspective would diminish and disappear. Rejoice that your soul essence has the vision and knowing to address any problem. The wisdom of your soul spans space and time. It can see energies, people, and situations being drawn to you before they arrive. It can see past patterns and events that are being repeated as common themes in your life. It knows the mission and purpose you have chosen. Choose to turn within and open to the insight of your Divine Self.

Meditation

Hold the symbol card to your heart (symbol facing your body) and ask your Divine Self to transfer the clearest and purest frequencies of the symbol to you. Ask that all resistance to seeing clearly be removed and transmuted.

Then choose to go within to connect with your soul essence through your heart. Ask to see the situation through the eyes of your soul. Ask for the clarity that rises above the circumstances and sees the Big Picture. Request that you be guided to align with your highest good.

Open to the impressions and guidance from the Source of your Being. The clearest vision you will ever obtain will be from your soul and from Source and the power and clarity of that sight lies within.

Color and Symbol Balancing

The primary color of this symbol is indigo, which energizes, clears and activates the brow chakra. Indigo helps to expand your inner vision and inner knowing by energizing the pituitary gland.

The secondary color of this symbol is purple, which helps you align with your spiritual mission and purpose.

The tertiary color is light lemon, which helps to clear and open the solar plexus chakra.

When projecting the vibration of the symbol, first see it on a stream of indigo light that infuses the head and brow chakra.

Visualize the brow chakra expanding and clearing. After the expansion of the brow feels complete, begin projecting the symbol's frequency on a river of purple light.

Let the purple light fill the head and then flow through the whole body. This will assist the individual in becoming sensitive to their spiritual nature. Hold the intention that the individual comes into alignment with the insight of their soul.

If necessary, a light lemon color can be visualized filling the solar plexus, to help clear blockages and emotional resistance to seeing the truth.

CARD #21
I Honor My Divine Magnificence

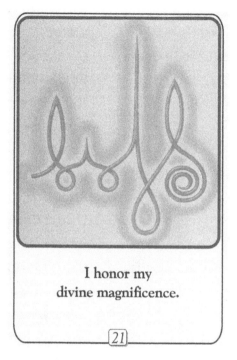

I honor my
divine magnificence.

21

AFFIRMATION

"I fully accept my Divine Essence and no longer hide from the magnificence I see in myself and others."

Insight

Know that beneath your personality, your Christos Nature, which connects you to all things, can free you to love and honor yourself. Looking outside of yourself for continual approval will always leave you unfulfilled. The worldly perception of who you are is subject to change. Your friends can have "bad days" and say less than kind words.

To build your sense of self-esteem upon worldly feedback is

CORRESPONDENCES

PRIMARY COLOR	Gold
SECONDARY COLOR	Turquoise
TERTIARY COLOR	Violet
METALS\CRYSTALS USED IN GRIDS:	Gold (metal)
	Golden Rutilated Quartz
	Golden Barite
	Turquoise
	Celestite
CHAKRAS CLEARED AND ALIGNED:	Crown Chakra
	Brow Chakra
	Throat Chakra
	Heart Chakra
MERIDIANS CLEARED AND ALIGNED:	Heart Meridian
	Small Intestine Meridian
	Urinary/Bladder Meridian
	Triple Warmer Meridian
	Gall Bladder Meridian
PRIMARY ELEMENTS REPRESENTED BY THE SYMBOL:	Ether/Fire/Air/Water

to construct your house on a weak and faulty foundation. Yet accepting your Divine Essence and grounding your self-acceptance in the Source and truth of your Being, is to base your self image upon your true magnificence.

Only through love and appreciation of yourself can you draw upon a well deep enough to continually express love to others. Embracing your Christos Nature and choosing to fully embody your truth is to honor your magnificence. This is not an expression of ego or pride, for such pride sees itself as apart from, and greater or lesser than others. When you perceive others through your Christos Nature, you see the Christos Nature in them. Becoming attuned to the unity of all souls results in a sense of equality.

Self-acceptance and self-love help you resist the temptation to give control over to the ego-personality which wants to judge, criticize, divide, and segregate. The ego-personality supports its existence through fear, guilt, shame, and anger. When you can honor and love the divinity of self and others, you move your center of focus away from the ego's belief in separation and shift it to a sense of unity, the foundational awareness of your soul.

The most significant way of stepping into your power is to fully express your love and magnificence from your heart and to operate from the Divine Source of your Being.

To do anything less is to see yourself as a victim of forces beyond your control. The position of the victim is one of powerlessness over thoughts, emotions, and life circumstances. Honoring your divinity, along with everyone else's, aligns you with the infinite grace and love of Source, as well as your inner wisdom and co-creative power.

The message and essence of this card, "I Honor my Divine Magnificence," may be difficult to accept if you hold onto the belief that you are not worthy of love, acceptance, or support. You can't love yourself if you are immersed in an internal dialogue of self-judgment.

Self-critical beliefs acquired in childhood can continue to color your perceptions of the world. Unfortunately, if you truly believe you are unworthy, you manifest life dramas to support that belief.

Choose to accept that you are worthy. Accept that as a child of God, of the stars, and of the universe, your magnificence is beyond all measure. Allow the unlimited love of Source to expand out from your heart and bless all that you know. As you truly believe you are divine, your magnificence will be shown to you through the Source of your Being.

Card for the Day

If your soul guided you to select this card today, it is time for you to honor your greatness, the miracle of your existence, and the uncountable blessings in your life. In all of creation, you are a unique expression of Source, a gift of Source to itself and there is none other exactly like you.

The essence of this symbol is about the full acceptance of your divinity. As you begin to use this symbol, any perception or denial of this truth will demand attention and all of your issues about being "less than" will come to the surface to be confronted. This is the natural process of release, which will bring about clarification and peace. Rejoice! There is nothing to fear and everything to gain.

Meditation

Mirror work is a powerful way to use this symbol. Do this meditation looking into a mirror. Study the color, form, and essence of the symbol. Find a quiet spot and bring your focus to your heart. Allow yourself to sink deep into your soul's essence. When you feel centered and aligned, bring the symbol card up to your heart with the symbol facing your body.

As you breathe in, visualize yourself drawing in the gold color of the symbol as well as the symbol's vibration. Feel the symbol's essence within your heart. Say to your Divine Self, "*Beloved Divine*

Self, I choose to fully embody the highest vibrational essence of this symbol within my Being and to honor my Divine Magnificence. I choose, as well, to love all parts of me that feel less than divine into unity. So be it. And so it is!"

Continue drawing in the symbol's color and vibration through your heart, allowing this energy to flow through your whole body.

Now, look into the mirror and directly into your own eyes. Begin repeating slowly, *"I honor my Divine Magnificence. I accept my Divine Magnificence."* As you continue to repeat these sentences, become conscious of any emotions or beliefs that might come up.

Allow these old energies and beliefs to be triggered. Love them. Then, choose to let them go. Visualize the gold light and the energy of the symbol dissolving them away.

It would be extremely empowering to continue this process, for perhaps ten minutes each day, until no resistance arises.

Color and Symbol Balancing

The primary color of the symbol is gold, the color of the Christos Ray. Gold assists in healing separation on all levels.

Turquoise, the secondary color, carries equal amounts of green and blue, thus serving as the bridging color between the heart chakra (green) and the throat chakra (blue). It also simultaneously activates both of these chakras.

Violet, the symbol's tertiary color, assists in the transmutation of lower emotional energies, such as fear and anger, to higher vibrational ones such as love. Violet also helps to open and activate the crown chakra.

Visualize the symbol's vibration first carried on a Violet Ray of light, filling and infusing the body. Set the intention as you do this that all resistance be transmuted to love.

Once it feels as if the energetic resistance to the symbol's essence has been cleared, move on to using the Turquoise Ray. See and feel the symbol's frequency carried on a current of turquoise light, filling particularly the heart and throat areas. Then imagine the turquoise color expanding out through the entire body, bringing it into harmony and balance.

Gold is the final suggested color. Visualize radiant gold light carrying the symbol's essence and filling the whole Being. Ask silently that the purest Christos light infuse every level of this magnificent child of God.

CARD #22

When My Mind Is at Rest, I Feel One with Source

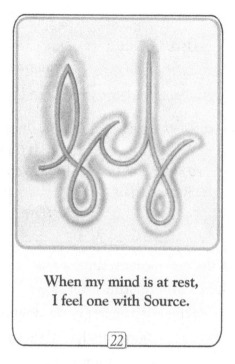

When my mind is at rest,
I feel one with Source.

[22]

AFFIRMATION

"I turn off my mind chatter and sink deep into the stillness, feeling my unity with Source."

Insight

The energy of this symbol helps you to let go of the parade of thoughts marching through your mind and to feel, through stillness, your connection with Source. It allows you to move to a level of awareness beyond thought where you feel yourself as an expression of All-That-Is.

When the constantly chattering mind, with all of its demands, fears, and warnings is allowed to rest, you can feel safe

CORRESPONDENCES	
PRIMARY COLOR	Cool Lake Blue
SECONDARY COLOR	Violet
TERTIARY COLOR	Peach
METALS\CRYSTALS USED IN GRIDS:	Blue Lace Agate
	Aquamarine
	Blue Quartz
	Larimar
CHAKRAS CLEARED AND ALIGNED:	Brow Chakra
	Throat Chakra
MERIDIANS CLEARED AND ALIGNED:	Triple Warmer Meridian
PRIMARY ELEMENTS REPRESENTED BY THE SYMBOL:	Air/Fire

and relaxed. In the peace that results, a space is created where you can sense unity with the Universal Flow.

Our Western civilization is left-brain dominated, placing reward and emphasis on logical, analytical thought and debate. However, an untrained mind, jumping from one need to another, can be a severe task master. It often leaves you viewing the world as fractured, unfriendly, and cold. Since the left-brain perceives the universe in separate pieces, it creates a belief in separation from Source and others.

The energetic essence of this symbol helps to balance the left and right hemispheres of the brain, shifting to a more equal sharing of cranial dominance. The symbol's energy assists in opening the crown chakra and activating the right brain. More life force (chi, ki) begins to move through the head, clearing up blockages in the left brain.

Although the symbol is energizing as described, the end result is to balance and harmonize the energy flow in the body, predominantly in the head. This initiates deep relaxation and movement to a level of awareness beyond thought; the mind chatter ceases and you can enter a place of stillness.

When you enter the stillness, you become open to your feeling nature, a right brain attribute. The longer you can stay in your feeling nature, the more sensitive you will become to every one and every thing in your energetic field. You will be able, for example, to walk in a forest and sense the pulsating bubble of life energetically created by the animals and plants living there.

The value of operating from our feeling nature is down played in our culture. Coming into balance involves promoting an equal dominance between our thinking and feeling capabilities, and our left and right brain hemispheres.

This symbol addresses the need to rest the analytical mind and relax in the space of silence where you can feel a deep abiding connection to Prime Creator and the Universal Field. This symbol opens the heart channel and assists in remembrance of your connection to the Great Spirit.

Card for the Day

If this card was selected, your Divine Self is suggesting it is a time to relax, to take it easy, and stop thinking so hard. Allow yourself to experience the peace that comes with the absence of thought. Take time to move into the stillness and embrace your own divinity. Shift your focus from your thinking nature to your feeling nature, and **Feel** your connection to the universe.

Meditation

Find a quiet place to meditate. Look at the symbol card for a few seconds, then bring it up to your heart (symbol facing your body).

Ask your Divine Self to transfer the vibrations of the symbol to all levels of your Being saying, "*Beloved Divine Self, I ask that the purest vibrations of this symbol be transferred to me. I ask that I experience the deep peace of No Thought. I choose to feel my connection with Source.*" Now, allow the energy of the symbol to become one with you. If you become aware of thoughts, let them float by like clouds without energizing them. Welcome the stillness and let it enfold you.

Color and Symbol Balancing

The symbol's primary color is a cool lake blue, which calms and relaxes the nervous system.

The symbol's secondary color is violet, a color which assists in opening the crown chakra and clearing any blocks in the flow of the life force.

The symbol's tertiary color is peach, which resonates with the essence of Universal Love, and helps keep the emotional body balanced and at peace.

Project the vibration of the symbol on a ray of cool lake blue light, allowing the blue light to fill and infuse the head. If it feels like blockages need to be cleared, project the symbol on a current of violet light, visualizing the violet light breaking up and dissolving all constrictions.

You may find yourself alternating back and forth between cool blue and violet, as layers of thought and emotions come to the surface to be released.

As a final step, you may want to wash the whole body in cool lake blue, followed by peach colored light.

CARD #23

I Choose to Experience Heaven on Earth

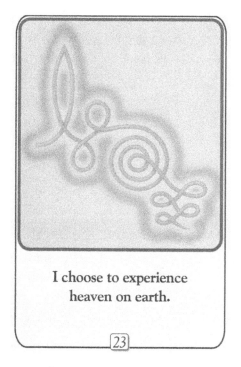

I choose to experience
heaven on earth.

[23]

AFFIRMATION

*"I experience the unity that springs from Source in
my relationship with all life."*

Insight

Experiencing Heaven on Earth involves walking in your divinity. "Heaven" is a state of consciousness, a state of being, of feeling grace and unity with All-That-Is. It is the full expression of your Christos nature. To experience this state on Earth is to embody this consciousness in all aspects of your life.

Experiencing Earth as Heaven involves the subtlest of shifts in perception where you finally see the unity beneath the illu-

CORRESPONDENCES

PRIMARY COLOR	Gold
SECONDARY COLOR	Soft Green
TERTIARY COLOR	Royal Blue
METALS\CRYSTALS USED IN GRIDS:	Gold (metal)
	Golden Topaz
	Dioptase
	Emerald
	Peridot
CHAKRAS CLEARED AND ALIGNED:	Crown Chakra
	Throat Chakra
	Heart Chakra
MERIDIANS CLEARED AND ALIGNED:	Heart Meridian
	Lung Meridian
	Heart Meridian
	Pericardium Meridian
	Triple Warmer Meridian
	Liver Meridian
PRIMARY ELEMENTS REPRESENTED BY THE SYMBOL:	Air/Fire/Earth

sion of separation.

Imagine rain falling on a large body of water like a lake. With each raindrop, small concentric waves move across the water, intersecting other waves, and forming a complex, ever-changing pattern on the surface.

The life you experience through your five senses is similar to the surface phenomenon of the lake where each wave seems distinct, unique and dynamic. Yet beneath the lake's surface is the massive body of water that supports the ripples on its surface. The physical forms (yourself, others, dogs, trees, buildings) appear separate yet are manifested from the formless Universal Field of Source. The Universal Field expresses itself through all things, and is the matrix from which everything arises and dissolves.

Seeing Source in all life is to acknowledge the unity from which all diversity springs. With this enhanced perspective, you can sense the order existing beneath the chaos on the surface, and you can find peace where you once experienced the pain of separation. A grace descends upon your life, as does a love for all expressions and forms. In the space of one breath you can discover that Heaven has always been on Earth.

The human species is multi-dimensional. This means you can choose to embrace the consciousness of some of the highest spiritual frequencies of the universe. Your physical form allows you to ground these energies into the densest vibrational levels of matter, thus granting you the capability to unify and bridge Earth and cosmos.

As you embody the love of your Christos nature, you also energetically anchor the vibration of love into the planet and into the world. When you discover Heaven within yourself, you simultaneously bring it to Earth. Each time this happens, the world is transformed.

Card for the Day

If you selected this card, your Divine Self is guiding you to transform your world by acknowledging the Heaven within yourself. Walking in love, you ground its vibration into the Earth with each step. As you sense Source beneath the surface of your relationships, in the wind, in the changing seasons, you will be able to sense Source in yourself. When you allow yourself to feel the Heaven within, you will see it manifest simultaneously in your outer world.

Meditation

In a secluded space, study the form, color, and energy of this symbol. Hold the symbol to your heart (symbol facing your body) and state: *"Beloved Divine Self, I choose to fully embody the highest essence and quality of the symbol into my Being. I choose to bring Heaven to Earth by honoring the divinity with myself. I now allow my highest spiritual qualities to unfold and manifest. So be it. And so it is!"*

Visualize the energy of this symbol entering your heart on a current of gold light. Feel the gold light flowing through every cell, tissue, organ, and gland in your body. Review in your mind the qualities you would most like to manifest (peace, love, courage). Feel yourself absorbing those qualities into your Being so they become an integral part of your life.

Color and Symbol Balancing

Gold, the symbol's primary color, strongly resonates with the Christ Ray. Gold activates and opens the heart chakra, crown chakra, and the chakras above the head. Gold helps heal fractures due to inner conflict in the energy bodies. It also assists in stabilizing, balancing, and grounding the life force energy.

Green, the symbol's secondary color, purifies and balances the physical body. It also helps to open and expand the heart.

Royal blue, the symbol's tertiary color, helps to open both the throat and brow chakras. Blue also assists in clearing the body of disease and discordant energy patterns.

It is recommended to use the green and gold colors when transmitting the symbol's frequency. Use the royal blue color only if it appears that the throat chakra is constricted.

Begin with green because of its cleansing qualities. Visualize the vibration of this symbol carried on the Green Ray, infusing the body at the deepest tissue layers. See the green light entering the heart and flooding the entire body. Set the intention that the green light melt and dissolve all blocks.

When it feels that all blocks have been cleared, follow with the Gold Ray. Imagine the symbol's energy carried on a radiant stream of gold light. As with the Forest Green Ray, direct the Gold Ray into the heart chakra and expand the light out through the body.

Fill the body with gold light and visualize the body as clear and bright as the sun. Choose that the symbol's frequency be integrated on all levels within the individual.

CARD #24
I Embrace Compassion

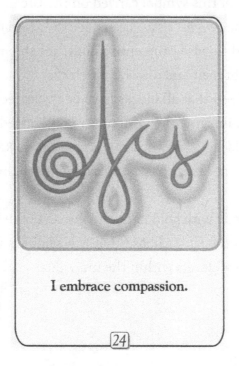

I embrace compassion.

[24]

AFFIRMATION

"I expand my heart, unifying with those from whom I have felt separated."

Insight

Your natural state, seen through the eyes of your soul, is one of unity with the world and everyone in your life. However, this natural state seems unnatural to your ego-personality. Compassion is the way back to the state of grace you left through judgment, division and fear. It is expressed in the Mayan phrase, *"You are another me."* It involves seeing yourself in another.

Compassion is living the understanding that your similari-

CORRESPONDENCES

PRIMARY COLOR	Pink
SECONDARY COLOR	Gold
TERTIARY COLOR	Silver
METALS\CRYSTALS USED IN GRIDS:	Rose Quartz
	Pink Kunzite
	Pink Tourmaline
	Peach Calcite
CHAKRAS CLEARED AND ALIGNED:	Heart Chakra
MERIDIANS CLEARED AND ALIGNED:	Lung Meridian
	Heart Meridian
PRIMARY ELEMENTS REPRESENTED	
BY THE SYMBOL:	Air/Fire

ties far outweigh the differences. When you comprehend that the crises you create in your life are orchestrated by your spirit to teach your personality lessons, it's easier to let go of the judgments you place on others. You begin to realize that everyone is doing the best they can. The deeper you sink into this awareness of unity, the easier it becomes to embrace compassion.

Compassion must start with self. It is difficult to have compassion for another when you don't have it for yourself. As you judge yourself, you cloud your perception of the world so that you have difficulty seeing anyone's true essence.

The judgments, criticisms, and doubts you place upon yourself are invariably projected out onto the world. When you let go of self-condemnation, it becomes easy to recognize yourself in another.

Perhaps the deepest expression of compassion is to see and respond to the divinity, the Christos Nature, in others. In equality, there is no condescending, no judgment: no right, wrong, better, greater. In seeing another's Divine Nature, the distortions you have in common fall away. What is left is the fabric of unity that has always been present, weaving the universe together.

Compassion is a state of grace that expands out from the heart. It is not an operation of the mind, but of the Spirit. When you connect to the soul of another from your own soul essence, you are uniting with their core, the Source of their Being. Your *"Sourceness"* is resonating with their *"Sourceness."* There can be no stronger bond of equality and love than communication at the soul level. In doing so, you dive beneath personality and judgment into the sea of At-One-Ment.

The deepest form of your compassion for another flows from your soul as you honor your own Divine Nature. The ability to see the holiness of another soul arises because you have accepted your own Divine Essence.

Card for the Day

If you selected this symbol card, you are blessed with the chance to offer compassion to another or to yourself. It is an opportunity to let go of all judgments, to love and to be loved. Go within and ask Spirit where compassion can best be expressed today. Is it with yourself or with another? Once you have received an answer, consider conducting the following meditation.

Meditation

Find a quiet and secluded place to study the symbol card. Focus on its color, form, and essence. Hold the card up to your heart chakra with the symbol facing your body. As you inhale, imagine drawing the pink energy of the card into your heart.

As you feel the essence of the symbol fill you, state the following, *"Beloved Divine Self, I ask that the purest qualities of compassion and acceptance become infused within me. Let me expand these qualities out, dissolving all separation I have ever felt. So be it. And so it is!"*

Visualize either yourself or another before you. If that individual is yourself, see yourself as radiant. Feel a pink bubble of light around your heart. Allow that bubble to expand, growing larger and larger. Let it first surround you and then the individual with whom you have felt separate.

Embrace that person and yourself in a bubble of pink unconditional love. Feel your bond of At-One-Ment with that individual. Know that individual is deserving and worthy of love.

Color and Symbol Balancing

Pink, the primary color of this symbol, resonates with the quality of unconditional love and works through the emotional aspect of the heart.

Gold, the symbol's secondary color, is representative of the Christ Ray. Silver, the tertiary color, is aligned with the Divine Mother aspect of acceptance and allowance.

It is suggested you begin by projecting the essence of the symbol on the Pink Ray. Visualize the pink light entering the heart and flowing through every part of the body. Imagine the essence of the symbol being infused into every cell. Hold the intention that compassion is embraced on all levels.

Ask for guidance as to whether to follow with the Gold or the Silver ray. Balance and harmony will best be achieved with:

1. Silver to bring in more of the feminine/lunar aspect, or

2. Gold to accent more of the masculine/solar aspect.

Feel the symbol's vibration carried on a current of either gold or silver light. Allow the light to fill and radiate out from the body. Again, hold the intention that compassion and love be felt and expressed on all levels.

CARD #25

I Am in Complete Harmony and Balance

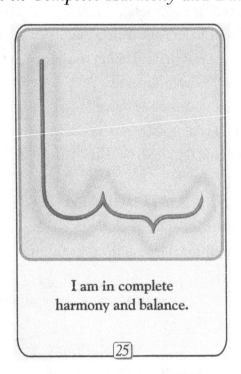

I am in complete
harmony and balance.

25

AFFIRMATION

*"I allow myself to be open, flexible, and in balance
by experiencing love from the Source of my Being."*

Insight

The essence of this symbol is flexibility through love. When
you walk on the deck of a rolling ship, you need to move in con-
cert with the wave motion to maintain your balance. You shift
your weight and move back to center if you feel yourself being
pushed off center.

Balance and harmony are dynamic states that exist within an
ever-changing field of action. The state of love creates the inner

CORRESPONDENCES

PRIMARY COLOR	Emerald Green
SECONDARY COLOR	Turquoise
TERTIARY COLOR	Silver
METALS\CRYSTALS USED IN GRIDS:	Dioptase
	Emerald
	Green Tourmaline
	Turquoise
	Green Apatite
	Silver (metal)
	Moonstone
CHAKRAS CLEARED AND ALIGNED:	Heart Chakra
	Throat Chakra
MERIDIANS CLEARED AND ALIGNED:	Spleen Meridian
	Heart Meridian
	Gall Bladder Meridian
	Liver Meridian
PRIMARY ELEMENTS REPRESENTED BY THE SYMBOL:	Earth

emotional flexibility which allows you to change at a moment's notice and to respond in harmony with the ever-shifting flow of life.

Walking in love, holding the state of love of self, others, and Source, manifests a powerful energy field that flows out from the center of your being and then back again. The energy field of love generated from a loving heart is ordered and coherent. It spins rapidly like a gyroscope. The stronger this field of love, the easier it is to remain in your center, your Divine Core Essence, where you experience balance and harmony. The imbalanced emotional states of fear, anger, bitterness, jealousy, and guilt cannot exist simultaneously within the field of unconditional love.

Love, representing the equal and opposite exchange of energies between the lover and the beloved, embodies the states of balance and harmony. You need not look outside of yourself for these qualities. Resolving your inner conflict creates the space of peace where you can feel safe enough to love yourself, others, and your Divine Source of Being. Out of this love, and through this love, you will discover its reflection of harmony and balance in your community and friends.

Remaining in harmony and balance also involves connecting with the energy flow and pulse of Nature by linking into the natural rhythms and cadences of the planet. The planet is constantly breathing; there are natural energy flows with the seasons, the weather, and the diurnal solar (day and night) cycles. Your biological body responds to these natural cycles of Mother Earth and needs to be in resonance with them to remain healthy and balanced.

The industrialized, electromagnetic environment (AM/FM radio, microwave) has many artificial energy cycles (e.g. 60 cycle alternating current) that shield and cut us off from the planet's natural rhythms. If you are feeling knocked off-center emotionally or physically, spending time in Nature (taking a walk in the forest or park) with the intention of reconnecting with the natural life force can be a valuable step to moving back into balance. Leaning against a tree and drawing the life force energy of the tree through you will bring energetic harmony to unsettled emotions.

Being centered and attuned with your heart engenders balance and harmony on every level of your life.

Card for the Day

If you have chosen this card, you may be moving into a new

level of balance and harmony within yourself and your relationships. Perhaps you may be feeling a little out-of-balance and out-of-sync. Or, maybe you don't feel aligned with some aspect of your life. If the imbalance is being reflected in your physical body, e.g., you're feeling sick, the harmony and vitality of Nature could assist you in moving back to your center.

One powerful technique is to stand or sit under a tree and, as you breathe in, imagine the green tree energy flowing in the crown of your head, moving down through your body, and out your feet as you exhale. Allow the rich green life force of the tree to clear all discord from your Being.

If the imbalance seems to exist on the emotional level, the following meditation is recommended.

Meditation

Study the color and shape of the symbol. Hold the symbol card to your heart (symbol facing your body) and say, "*Beloved Divine Self, I now choose to absorb the purest qualities of balance and harmony represented by this symbol. I choose to come into complete alignment with my Divine Core Essence and express this centeredness in all levels of my life.*"

Visualize the emerald green color and the energy of the symbol flowing into your heart, then out through your whole body. Allow yourself to come into resonance with the pulse of the universe.

Color and Symbol Balancing

Emerald green, the primary color of this symbol, balances and purifies the physical body as well as opens the heart chakra.

Turquoise, the symbol's secondary color, acts as a bridge between the heart and throat chakras; it symbolically merges the sky (blue) and Earth (green) energies.

Silver, the symbol's tertiary color, resonates with the Divine Feminine, the Divine Mother Ray, and enhances the qualities of allowance and acceptance.

When projecting the symbol's vibration, see it carried on a stream of emerald green light. Visualize the emerald green light flowing into the heart chakra and then expanding out through the entire body. As the green light radiates through every cell, tissue, and organ, imagine it flushing away all resistance and darkness.

If it appears that the individual is having difficulty in expressing him or her self or actualizing his or her dreams (walking their talk), activation of the throat and heart chakras with turquoise light can help. Imagine the symbol's essence carried on the Turquoise Ray, melting away blocks in these chakras.

Silver is a color of balance and to be most effective, it is recommended that it be used after the clearing performed with the colors of green and turquoise. Visualize the symbol's vibration being carried on the Silver Ray, filling the body and auric field, and anchoring the person solidly to Earth.

CARD #26
I Clear All within Me That Is Not of the Light

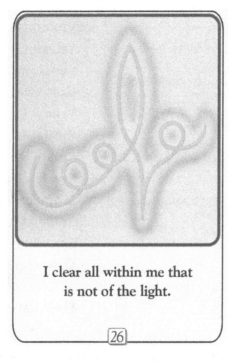

I clear all within me that
is not of the light.

26

AFFIRMATION

"I choose to transmute all fear, anger, bitterness, jealousy, and guilt within me to light."

Insight

This symbol carries the intention to clear and transmute the emotional energies that create heaviness and resistance within your being (e.g., fear, anger, guilt, grief). It initiates clearing by removing the cap or lid held over the suppressed and repressed emotions, allowing the dense emotional baggage to be lifted. The clearing is accomplished through the high spiritual vibrancy of the soul which can assist in cutting through illusion and drama.

CORRESPONDENCES

PRIMARY COLOR	Bright Yellow
SECONDARY COLOR	Orange
TERTIARY COLOR	Violet
METALS\CRYSTALS USED IN GRIDS:	Yellow Citrine
	Sunstone-Heliolite
	Gold (metal)
	Yellow Tiger Eye
	Rutilated Quartz
CHAKRAS CLEARED AND ALIGNED:	Solar Plexus Chakra
	Sexual Chakra
MERIDIANS CLEARED AND ALIGNED:	Stomach Meridian
	Spleen Meridian
	Small Intestine Meridian
	Liver Meridian
PRIMARY ELEMENTS REPRESENTED	
BY THE SYMBOL:	Fire/Water

Emotions have often been described as energy in motion, each with a different frequency and vibration. Those emotions which we call "negative," such as fear, anger, and guilt, have a low frequency and can be experienced as heavy, similar to a dense mass in the body. "Positive" emotions, such as love and joy, have a high frequency and feel light, weightless, and free of mass.

The emotions of love, joy, and bliss, carry a strong energetic charge which can clear and dissolve the lower frequency emotions in the body. In short, if the love is great enough, it can transmute all fear. The unconditional love of the soul, when fully expressed in form, clears all that is not like itself.

This symbol works through an alignment with your spiritual essence which could be thought of as the clearest and highest frequency of your *"Beingness"* on Earth. When you begin to align with the Core of Your Being, the lower frequency emotions of fear, rage and sadness are cleared in the purity of your spiritual essence.

This process usually begins with the dissolving of the emotional layer which has been keeping feelings hidden in the subconscious. Once the lid is removed, the suppressed or repressed emotions come to the conscious surface to be recognized, addressed and surrendered.

When this process is initiated, it is important to be okay with yourself and the emotions you are feeling. Consider them old energy. Allow yourself to experience the emotions and choose to clear them forever from your life. If you place a judgment on yourself or on the emotions you are experiencing, you are creating yet another cap of repression. Think of yourself as an open tube, through which the old emotions can flow.

Allow yourself to feel the emotional charge with the realization that it is an old program and old energy that does not reflect who you are. Choose, as well, that as you feel the old emotional charge, it will be cleared forever from your life.

Acknowledge that the old emotion and belief that served you once, no longer serves you now. Thank the "old energy" and let it go. As you experience the "emotional charge," feel it flow out of your root chakra like escaping smoke.

Remember, the Real You extends far beyond your emotions. Just as a computer is not its software, you are not your old emotional patterns. Choose to clear forever all of the emotionally charged programs that are keeping you from expanding into love.

Card for the Day

If you selected this symbol, you are being given the opportunity to clear away old emotional energy that has been hindering your expansion. It's time to clean house, knowing you will feel lighter and better at the end of the process. The following meditation is highly recommended.

Meditation

Study the symbol, its shape and colors. Hold the symbol card to your heart (symbol facing your body) chakra and ask, "*Beloved, Divine Self, I ask that the purest vibrations of this symbol fill my Being. I choose to clear and transmute all emotional energies that continue the illusion that I am separate and* (angry, fearful, lonely, sad, bitter, or whatever is appropriate). *I choose to clear and transmute these old energies to Light and Love forever. So be it. And so it is!*"

Visualize violet light flowing down over you and through you, as if you were sitting beneath a waterfall. Choose that the violet light clear all old energy patterns from your cells and tissues. Sit for a while, allowing the clearing to take place. Then, imagine the bright yellow color from the symbol entering your body and filling all the voids and spaces left behind when the old energies were cleared. Feel yourself radiating the color of bright yellow sunlight from your entire Being.

Color and Symbol Balancing

Yellow, the primary color of this symbol, assists in opening the solar plexus chakra, where you carry the majority of your low-grade emotional energies. Yellow also clarifies and harmonizes the mental body.

The symbol's secondary color, orange, expands the second (sexual) chakra, the energy center which you draw upon for your creative expressions. People often close their second chakra when they have fear about extending themselves forward into something new.

Violet, the tertiary color of this symbol, carries the Seventh Ray ability to transmute all low frequency emotions to high vibratory Light.

It is recommended that the symbol's frequency be projected first on a current of violet light. Imagine the violet light flowing through all the chakras, dissolving any blockages. Violet is a powerful color for purifying and clearing old emotional complexes.

The symbol's primary color, yellow, would be the next suggested color to broadcast the symbol's energy. Visualize yellow light, as bright as the sun, radiating out from the solar plexus, sweeping through the entire body. Spend some time in the solar plexus area allowing the yellow light and the symbol to penetrate deeply and burn away all resistance.

Use the orange light to carry the symbol's vibration if the individual seems to have low vitality and appears listless.

Card #27
I Live Only in the Eternal Now

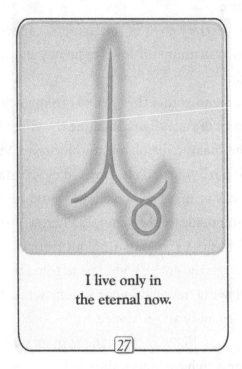

I live only in
the eternal now.

27

Affirmation

"I live in the eternal moment of my Divine Being."

Insight

When you let go of your past and future fears, the eternal present expands to fill your being. Within this eternal moment, you are aligned with the flow of the universe.

Recent research of the left and right brain hemispheres suggests that they perceive the world differently. The left-brain lives within a linear sense of time, creating a past, present, and future time flow. The right-brain lives only in the ever-present moment, unifying all elements of time into the singularity of the Now.

CORRESPONDENCES

PRIMARY COLOR	Electric Blue
SECONDARY COLOR	Forest Green
TERTIARY COLOR	Golden Yellow
METALS\CRYSTALS USED IN GRIDS:	Aqua Aura
	Celestite
	Blue Kyanite
	Blue Sapphire
CHAKRAS CLEARED AND ALIGNED:	Throat Chakra
	Heart Chakra
MERIDIANS CLEARED AND ALIGNED:	Small Intestine Meridian
	Triple Warmer Meridian
PRIMARY ELEMENTS REPRESENTED BY THE SYMBOL:	Ether/Fire

Your left-brain, the seat of logic, discriminates and judges your life, seeing the universe in terms of pieces, parts, boundaries, and limitations. The right-brain perceives the universe in unity, as a gestaltic whole; all parts seen in relationship to each other within a larger unifying pattern.

Thus, the sense of yourself as expansive, whole and at one with all things arises out of the right-brain's perceptions of the Eternal Now. "*Living in the moment*" occurs when your left- and right-brain perceptions of the world move into balance.

The Eternal Now is your point of liberation from the past and future. You often tenaciously hold onto past traumas, re-energizing them again and again, and experiencing them again and again. Forgiving yourself, forgiving everyone that you felt hurt you or did you wrong, helps dissolve these dysfunctional memories and programs. The decisions you made about yourself and others during these past traumas become dysfunctional belief systems which you constantly project into the future, resulting in a future that is a continuation of the past. Therefore, you continue to draw your fears to you. When you stop re-living the past or projecting your fears into the future, you will discover the power, wonder, and magic of the Eternal Now, the singular present.

In truth, only the present exists. What you think of as the past is but distorted memories stored electrochemically within your Being. What you perceive as the future is an extension of your present belief systems. Only the present, the Eternal Now, the infinite oneness, exists. It is here, in the Eternal Now, that all of the power of creation exists.

Living in the Eternal Now is fully experiencing the beauty around you without thinking about the past or worrying about the future. It is immersing yourself fully in the tastes and colors of the food you are eating without distracting yourself at the same time by reading a book or watching TV.

It is also realizing that right now, in this moment, you have the power to completely change your life through your choices and intentions rather than blaming your conditions on the past.

Ultimately, living in the infinite now involves fully experiencing one's unity with the Source of one's Being.

Card of the Day

If you selected this card, you may be spending a lot of your personal time and energy focusing on the past or worrying about the future. Choose instead to immerse yourself in the Eternal Now.

Take a moment to review all the wondrous things that exist in your life. Go for a walk in nature, absorbing the colors, sounds and textures of the living world. Hug a tree, feel the form of a rock, walk barefoot in the grass. Allow yourself to be aware of all that is sacred and holy in your life. Realize that your vast and infinite power to alter the course of your life rests in the Eternal Present. In this infinite moment, the beliefs and intentions you focus on will quickly manifest into form.

Choose intentions which are awe-inspiring, expansive and joy-filled. Forgive your past, forgive your parents, forgive your former spouse, forgive yourself. Let go of the trauma of the past and step into the power and beauty of the Holy Instant.

Meditation

The Eternal Now is most profoundly felt in the stillness of your inner being. In a place away from distraction, study the symbol. Allow your breathing to be slow, deep, and rhythmic. Bring the symbol up to your heart with the symbol facing your body. With each in-breath, picture the electric blue color of the symbol flowing into your heart and body. Say silently to yourself, "*I now choose to embody the purest essence of this symbol, experiencing the Eternal Now. So be it. And so it is.*"

Visualize yourself standing before a cool blue lake representing your soul essence. Step into the water. Surrender! Sink deep into the waters of your soul. Imagine and feel yourself sinking deeper and deeper into the stillness and peace of your inner Being. Allow the ever-present moment to expand gracefully and fill the space once occupied by the thoughts of your busy day.

Color and Symbol Balancing

The primary color of this symbol is electric blue, the color most often associated with Archangel Michael. The electric blue of Michael carries the vibration that cuts through the illusion of the past, the polarity conflicts of the present, and the projected fears of the future. With the veils removed, you can experience the Eternal Now.

When projecting the vibration of the symbol to someone, see high intensity electric blue light directed out of your hand. Feel the symbol's frequency carried on the electric blue stream of light. Visualize the electric blue light flooding the person's auric field and form. Set the intention that the light transmutes all issues keeping the individual from experiencing the Eternal Now, the infinite present.

After it feels as if all blockages have been cleared, continue by projecting the symbol's frequency on a Forest Green Ray of light. Allow the forest green light to infuse all levels of the recipient's being (cells, tissues, organs, glands). The forest green color will help bring balance and harmony to the physical and emotional bodies.

The symbol's tertiary color is golden yellow. Project this color into someone's solar plexus if he or she is expressing feelings of powerlessness or victimization. Visualize the golden yellow light as bright as the sun. Visualize the light burning away all blocks keeping the person from living in the Eternal Now.

CARD #28

I Choose the Completion of My Desire

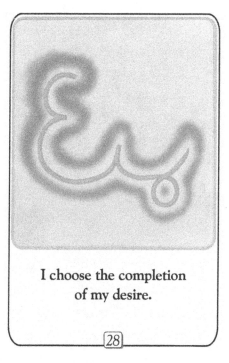

I choose the completion
of my desire.

28

AFFIRMATION

*"I choose fulfilment of my desire and I step off the
fence of indecision and fear."*

Insight

The essence of this card helps you to jump off the fence of indecision and make a choice to manifest a goal. We often bind and invest tremendous energy in unresolved issues and conflicts. Once we choose completion of a goal, we unlock and take back the power we had focused on our inner battle.

Indecision arises out of an inner conflict between opposing beliefs and emotions ("Yes, I can do it" versus "No, I can't do it.)

CORRESPONDENCES

PRIMARY COLOR	Bright Lemon Yellow
SECONDARY COLOR	Light Purple
TERTIARY COLOR	Sky Blue
METALS\CRYSTALS USED IN GRIDS:	Yellow Calcite
	Yellow Citrine
	Gold Topaz
	Rutilated Quartz
CHAKRAS CLEARED AND ALIGNED:	Solar Plexus Chakra
MERIDIANS CLEARED AND ALIGNED:	Spleen Meridian
	Kidney Meridian
PRIMARY ELEMENTS REPRESENTED BY THE SYMBOL:	Air/Earth/Water

The energy oscillates between one polarity and the other and nothing gets resolved or accomplished.

When you choose completion, you are choosing to "go for it" to press through the indecision, to move through the fear and to be willing to look at and address the unresolved issues which have kept you in a stalemate. Once the choice for completion is fully made, the universe aligns with your intention and supports its manifestation. All the resources you need are drawn to you.

When you become clear on every level of your life about what you want to experience and create, tremendous power is unleashed to manifest your desires. However, if you are caught in the cross currents of old conflicts, you often don't move into the choice for completion. Your left brain personality can easily perpetuate reasonable arguments on either side of an issue, keeping you from coming to resolution. The "*I Choose the Completion of My Desire*" symbol carries a vibration which can assist you in stepping out of indecision and moving forward.

There is an easy process for stepping off the fence. It involves realizing that your Source essence is your access to infinite wisdom. When you turn within to the Source of your Being for guidance, every question is answered from the highest state of knowing.

Once you ask to receive guidance and then step into the vision of your wish fulfilled, you actually initiate movement towards the goal's completion. For when you feel joy and blessings because you have received your intention, your vision has already manifested energetically. It's merely a matter of time before it appears in the physical. The intention to manifest your goal will re-order, shift, clear and dissolve many lower priority issues.

"Whatever you can do, or dream you can, begin it.
Boldness has genius, power and magic in it. Begin it now."

—Goethe

Card for the Day

If you have been guided to this symbol, you may be feeling stuck or on the fence in some part of your life. Know that as soon as you choose completion and begin to take the appropriate action, the universe will fully support you. Once you choose to accomplish your goal, tremendous forces are set in motion on the higher dimensional level to manifest your desired outcome.

Meditation

In a still and quiet place, bring your focus to your heart and feel your connection with the Source of your Being. Ask your Divine Self how you can reach completion of your unresolved issue or problem. Ask to be shown a vision of the action to be taken and a vision of your goal fully manifested.

Once you receive an answer, hold the symbol card to your

heart (symbol facing your body) and state: "*Beloved Divine Self, I choose to move to completion; I now wish to embody the highest vibrational quality of this symbol in my Being, assisting me in the manifestation of my intention. So be it. And so it is!*"

As you inhale, visualize yourself drawing in the vibration of the symbol into your heart and being. When you feel infused with the symbol's energy, clearly hold the vision of your intention accomplished. Feel the joy, grace, and satisfaction that comes with its manifestation.

Color and Symbol Balancing

Bright lemon is the primary color of this symbol; it assists in opening, purging, and purifying the solar plexus chakra. Traumas and fear of taking risks or stepping forward are most likely to be held in the solar plexus.

Light purple is the secondary color and resonates with high spiritual ideals and goals.

Sky blue, the symbol's tertiary color, assists in clearing the throat chakra so you can speak your truth.

In the majority of cases, the solar plexus chakra is the energetic focal point where you will want to introduce the symbol's vibration. Visualize the symbol's essence carried on a current of bright lemon light, entering and clearing the solar plexus chakra. If you psychically detect areas of darkness in the solar plexus, imagine the darkness being burned away by the intense lemon light.

When the solar plexus chakra feels fully charged, move up to the throat chakra. Project the symbol's vibration on a ray of sky blue light into the throat chakra, infusing that area completely. Use the color purple if the recipient appears blocked in the crown or brow chakras.

CARD #29

In Unity, All Things Are Possible

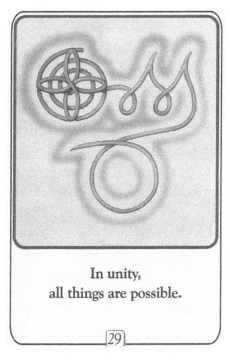

In unity,
all things are possible.

29

AFFIRMATION

"My Consciousness of At-One-Ment allows me to rise above the belief that I am separate from what I desire. Being unified with my vision, I manifest it in my life."

Insight

Through love, the lover is united with the beloved. Love is an expression of unification, of the embracing and the dissolving of fear and separation. In the love of self, of God, of the world, and others, all things are possible.

If you feel you "need" or "want" something, you are coming from the belief that you are separate from what you desire. This

CORRESPONDENCES

PRIMARY COLOR	Emerald Green
SECONDARY COLOR	Violet
TERTIARY COLOR	Purple
METALS\CRYSTALS USED IN GRIDS:	Diapotase
	Green Tourmaline
	Emerald
	Green Jade
	Amythest
CHAKRAS CLEARED AND ALIGNED:	Heart Chakra
	Crown Chakra
MERIDIANS CLEARED AND ALIGNED:	Heart Meridian
	Urinary/Bladder Meridian
PRIMARY ELEMENTS REPRESENTED BY THE SYMBOL:	Fire/Water

makes manifestation difficult—if not impossible. However, if you love yourself and your vision, the most natural state of bonding occurs between your vision and yourself, and you magnetize and love your heart's desire into existence.

You are already unified with all things and all possibilities, and you have the latent power to bring all potentialities into form through love and focus. Beliefs such as "it's impossible" and "I can't do it" perpetuate the concept of limitation when, in truth, there is no limitation. You are bonded with everything that has existed, exists, or ever shall exist. The unified field of consciousness connects all parts of the universe, on all levels. The deeper you allow yourself to feel the connection with the Source of your Being, the stronger you will sense the bond of love that binds you to the stars.

When you feel a strong sense of unity with the universe, you begin creating synchronicity in your life. Synchronicity occurs when fortuitous coincidences manifest in your reality from the Great Unknown.

You think of a friend you have not heard from in a year and she calls. You don't know where to find a specific fact and a book falls off your library shelf, opening to the exact page with the necessary information. You start planning a trip abroad and just happen to bump into someone, whom you have never met before, who has visited all locations you want to visit.

These "synchronistic" coincidences which appear to be happy coincidences are, in fact, arranged in the Universal Field behind the scenes. Synchronistic events become more common in your life as you love yourself and approach the conscious knowing state that you are unified with All-That-Is.

Card for the Day

If you chose this card, focus on the truth that as you love and allow your vision to "feel" real, the unifying and bonding power of love will bring it into physical existence. Acknowledge, deep within your being that you have universal and unlimited connections. And through the cosmic web of energy and consciousness, *"all you had hoped for"* or *"dreamed of,"* exists within the infinite constellation of possibilities.

Be prepared and watch for synergistic events as the resources of your vision are drawn to you in the manifestation process. Affirm that *"miracles are possible."* Affirm as well that *"you are safe," "you like yourself," "you love yourself," "you trust yourself,"* and *"you trust the Source of your Being."*

These affirmations help dissolve the sense of separation and assist you in reconnecting with and riding the Universal Flow.

Rejoice and know that the more passionately you love life, the more you will discover that what you though was impossible becomes possible.

Meditation

Select a goal you would like to create in your life. Select one that doesn't involve another person so your creation process does not involve manipulation or interference with another.

Visualize that this goal has already manifested. Step into it. Paint your visualization with as much detail, color, sound and smell as you can. Allow yourself to feel the emotions of your goal fully manifested: feel the joy, satisfaction, and sense of completion.

When you have a clear, crisp visualization in mind, study the color and form of the symbol. Bring the symbol up to your heart with the symbol facing your body. Imagine the emerald green color of the symbol radiating from the symbol and entering your heart. Allow your body to come into balance as it fills with the emerald green light.

Silently say to yourself, "*I now embody the highest quality and essence of this symbol. I sense my unlimited potential arising from my connection with Source. I know, since I am one with all things, that all things are possible. So be it. And so it is.*"

As you feel the energy of the symbol and intention flowing through you, bring your focus back to your visualization. Embrace it, live it. Know that as you see it in your mind's eye and feel the positive emotions, your goal has already begun to take form.

Color and Symbol Balancing

Emerald green is the primary color of this symbol. The color assists in the opening of the heart chakra, bringing balance within the body of the cosmic and Earth energies.

Violet, the secondary color, and purple, the tertiary color, both catalyze purification, clearing, and alignment with the highest spiritual frequencies. Violet and purple activate the crown chakra and higher chakras above the body.

If you sense blocks or constrictions in your client's chakras and energy bodies, it would be best to start with either violet or purple. Visualize the symbol's essence carried on a current of violet or purple light, entering the blocks and dissolving them.

Ask Spirit to guide you to the blocks that represent your client's resistance to manifesting their heart's desire. Run the color through his/her entire body until it appears clear and pristine in your mind's eye.

Once the body feels energetically open, begin projecting the symbol's vibration on a stream of emerald green light. Visualize the emerald green light filling the heart area and expanding out through the whole body. Feel your client's heart opening to the greater flow of Universal Love.

Ask your clients to choose to experience unity and harmony, knowing that from the place of unity all things are possible. When they have moved to a place of peace, suggest that they visualize their wish already fulfilled, to visualize their desire fully manifested.

CARD #30

I Now Welcome the Manifestation of My Desire

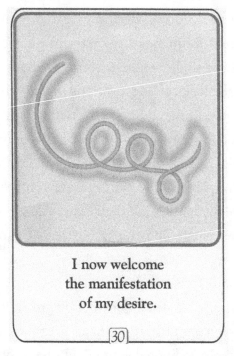

I now welcome
the manifestation
of my desire.

30

AFFIRMATION

*"Having chosen my intention, I welcome it with open
arms and an open heart."*

Insight

One of the most important aspects of conscious manifestation is the act of loving and welcoming what you choose into existence. In the act of welcoming, you are an open vessel for that which you desire.

We possess the power of manifestation. Indeed, we are manifesting our thoughts and beliefs all the time. However, the manifestation of our reality is usually, for the most part, a

---

CORRESPONDENCES

PRIMARY COLOR	Emerald Green
SECONDARY COLOR	Turquoise
TERTIARY COLOR	Forest Green
METALS\CRYSTALS USED IN GRIDS:	Green Tourmaline
	Green Jade
	Emerald
	Green Apatite
CHAKRAS CLEARED AND ALIGNED:	Heart Chakra
MERIDIANS CLEARED AND ALIGNED:	Heart Meridian
	Kidney Meridian
PRIMARY ELEMENTS REPRESENTED	
BY THE SYMBOL:	Fire/Water

---

subconscious process.

If you are uncomfortable with your life, you have probably manifested subconscious beliefs and programs about lack, unworthiness and low self-esteem.

On the other hand, with focused intention and creative imagination (emotionally rich visualizations), you can begin to creatively choose and manifest that which is in alignment with your heart's desire.

There are four basic steps to manifesting your desires with grace:

1. Set your intention. Visualize with clarity that which you desire.

2. Step into your visualization. Experience it happening now.

3. Feel and live your vision with all of your five senses. See it, touch it, taste it, smell it and hear it happening.

4. Surrender the details of how it is to manifest to Source and your unconscious mind. Simultaneously welcome, allow and accept the manifestation without doubt.

For example, let us suppose you need to find a new residence. First, decide how much space you need. Include all of your other requirements (number of rooms, apartment or house, city or country, location). Be as clear and specific as possible. Write it down.

Second, visualize yourself living, playing, and working in your new home/apartment, and that it fulfills all of your desires.

Third, visualize your fully manifested dream using all your senses. See your wish fulfilled, hear it, smell it, taste it and touch it. Let your heart sing with joy.

Fourth, act as if God were handling all the details for you. Welcome the arrival of your new home with confidence by going window shopping for furnishings.

The act of welcoming, then, is the joyous opening to receive and create the space for the manifestation. Imagine yourself welcoming your manifestation as you would welcome your best friend to your home. You stand with open arms, greeting your friend with pleasure. With gladness in your heart, you accept your friend into your embrace.

Welcoming your intention into manifestation is greeting its arrival with joy, accepting it into your embrace, loving it into existence and acting as if it has already happened.

The welcoming is done in faith and trust. All doubt and fear has been dissolved. You welcome your creation into form in love, knowing it will appear.

Card for the Day

If you selected this card, there is a goal or intention that can be welcomed into your life.

What is your heart's desire at this time? How would you feel and act if you knew with certainty that your heart's desire were coming your way? Know that you are closer than you might think to obtaining it.

Embrace the visualized desire in your heart, welcoming it home with the same passion that you would welcome the arrival of your best friend. See your heart's desire on your doorstep. Anticipate its manifestation with excitement.

Meditation

Choose a goal that you would like to draw into your life now. Visualize it as fully manifested. Follow the guidelines described in this symbol's *Insight* section for the visualization process. Create the visualization with clarity and detail, and allow yourself to feel your heart's desire is fulfilled.

Once you have selected your visualization, take time to study the symbol. In a space away from noise and distraction, bring the symbol up to your heart with the symbol facing your body. Feel a stream of emerald green light flowing from the symbol into your heart and every part of your body. Choose to sink deep into the peace and stillness of your inner being.

State to yourself, *"I choose to embody the purest essence of this symbol"* and *"I now welcome my heart's desire into my life with an open heart. So be it. And so it is."*

Embrace your vision with love.

See and experience your goal as present and filling you with joy.

Color and Symbol Balancing

Emerald green is the primary color of this symbol. This color helps to open the heart chakra and supports "the loving" of your desire into form.

Turquoise, the symbol's secondary color, is a color resulting from the combination of green and blue. It carries some of the antiseptic and cooling properties of blue. Turquoise also activates the thymus gland and assists in bridging the heart and throat chakras.

Forest green, the symbol's tertiary color, is a more Earthy green and like "emerald" expands the heart. It also brings balance to the physical body.

If your friend appears to have an immune system that is being challenged (for example, has a cold or flu virus) begin with the color turquoise. Visualize the essence of the symbol carried on a stream of turquoise light that fills the thymus gland, heart, lungs, and whole body. Feel the color and symbol penetrate deeply into the body tissues.

If guided, follow turquoise with forest green, a color which can assist the body in moving into harmony and health. Again, see and feel the symbol's forest green color soaking into the body's cells, organs, and glands. Choose, as you do this, that your client manifests health and peace.

The symbol's primary color, emerald green, is perhaps the most powerful color to use when projecting the symbol's essence. Visualize emerald green light flowing into your client's heart chakra and their heart opening slowly like the petals of a lotus. Know that, as they expand their heart to receive the ever present love in their Divine Core, they will welcome their dreams into their life with ease.

CARD #31

I Allow Abundance on All Levels into My Life

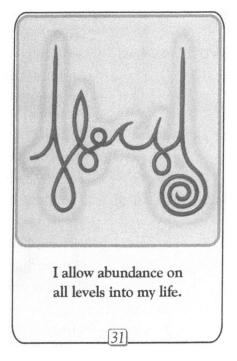

I allow abundance on
all levels into my life.

[31]

AFFIRMATION

"I feel At-One with everything and as a result, want nothing. I allow my natural state of abundance to fill me and bless every aspect of my life."

Insight

Experiencing abundance in your life is just allowing this natural state to exist, without imposing any conditions. When you feel at-one with everything, then all your "needs" and "wants" melt away. When you know you are an extension of the universe, it is difficult to feel you are lacking anything. Every issue of lack arises out of a belief in separation from Source and

CORRESPONDENCES

PRIMARY COLOR	Purple
SECONDARY COLOR	Soft Green
TERTIARY COLOR	Gold
METALS\CRYSTALS USED IN GRIDS:	Amethyst
	Sugilite-Luvulite
	Selenite
	Herkimer Diamond
CHAKRAS CLEARED AND ALIGNED:	Crown Chakra
	Brow Chakra
	Heart Chakra
MERIDIANS CLEARED AND ALIGNED:	Large Intestine Meridian
	Heart Meridian
	Urinary/Bladder Meridian
	Pericardium Meridian
	Triple Warmer Meridian
PRIMARY ELEMENTS REPRESENTED BY THE SYMBOL:	Fire/Air/Water

the Universal Supply.

Since abundance is your natural state of grace, you have to expend a great deal of energy to maintain the illusion of scarcity. You need to continually reinforce beliefs of lack, which hold fear in place and block the flow. Any fear of loss or of losing control can constrict your sense of abundance.

Thus, abundance is not something to strive for; it is more a matter of clearing your fears and returning to your natural state of grace. Surrendering your need to control will release the blocks. Choosing to embrace your unity with all things will dispel the sense of isolation.

Abundance is truly a state of mind. When you can love yourself, you can feel abundant—no matter what the circumstances. As you clear your inner conflict and experience peace, you also experience abundance. It is difficult to feel a deep sense of peace and simultaneously believe you are poor.

This symbol assists one in opening to the Universal Flow. You are surrounded by abundance. All you need to do is surrender, drop your defenses, and allow it to flood into your life.

"Love of Self" and feeling worthy are the core and fundamental states of Being that will open the doors to abundance. This symbol helps to align with your Christos Nature and the energy of love, which is the energetic substrate of the universe. It assists in resonating with the love at the Source of your Being and feeling your worthiness as a child of God. We are all equal in the eyes of Spirit, and the Universal Field of Consciousness makes abundance available to all who are open to receive it.

Card for the Day

If you have selected this card, take a moment to reflect on the friends, love, and beauty in your life. Take time to give thanks for everything in your life that fills your heart with joy. The deeper your sense of gratitude, the wider the portals will open to the abundance of the universe. Feeling blessed allows blessings to manifest in your outer world.

Meditation

Sit in a quiet spot. Study the symbol and attune to its essence. Hold the symbol card to your heart (symbol facing your body) and ask your Divine Self, "*Beloved Divine Self, I ask that the purest vibrations of this symbol be transferred to all levels of my Being. I ask to be brought into alignment with the infinite love* and abundance of the universe. So be it. And so it is!'"

Picture, in your mind, everything in your life for which you now feel blessed: your best friends, your pets, your hobbies, your freedom. After honoring the abundance already present begin picturing yourself allowing even more abundance to fill your life.

Note: Do not come from a space of needing or wanting something, rather, see yourself already connected to your desired manifestations. See and feel yourself experiencing the Universal Flow in your life. Step into your wish fulfilled, and allow yourself to sing joyfully for its coming manifestation in form.

Color and Symbol Balancing

Purple is the primary color of this symbol. It helps to open the crown chakra and clear resistance within your energy field.

Green, the symbol's secondary color, expands the heart and brings the physical body into harmony and balance.

Gold, the symbol's tertiary color, is the color of the Christ Ray. Gold assists you in acknowledging your unity with All-That-Is.

First project the symbol's vibration on a current of purple light. Visualize the Purple Ray filling the head, opening the crown chakra, and burning away any darkness in the body.

Then, project the symbol's essence on the Green Ray, infusing the heart with this color. Visualize the heart chakra expanding as it is filled with green light.

Lastly, feel the symbol's vibrations carried on the Gold Christ Ray. See gold light pouring into the crown and heart chakras, filling the body until the light overflows. Silently, affirm that the gold light represents the client's natural state of abundance.

CARD #32
Not My Will, Lord, But Thine

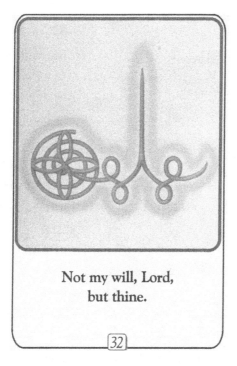

Not my will, Lord,
but thine.

32

AFFIRMATION

"I surrender and let go of my personal needs and immerse myself in the Source of my Being."

Insight

This card addresses the surrender of the small ego to the greater will of God. It is not letting go to some force or agent outside of you. Rather, it is surrendering to your own True Nature, your True Self. It is a shift in perspective from the micro to the macro, from the exclusive to the inclusive, from the many illusory personality desires that drive you, to resting in your Divine Being.

In Western culture, we are conditioned by our society, by

CORRESPONDENCES

PRIMARY COLOR	Gold
SECONDARY COLOR	Yellow
TERTIARY COLOR	Violet
METALS\CRYSTALS USED IN GRIDS:	Gold (metal)
	Gold Citrine
	Gold Topaz
	Amythest
CHAKRAS CLEARED AND ALIGNED:	All chakras with an emphasis on the solar plexus chakra
MERIDIANS CLEARED AND ALIGNED:	All meridians with an emphasis on the kidney meridian
PRIMARY ELEMENTS REPRESENTED BY THE SYMBOL:	Fire/Air/Ether/ Water/Earth

the media, and by our peers, to desire status through position, money, and material possessions. Perhaps all of these desires are rooted in beliefs of lack—that what we require is outside of us and that we are less than whole or complete without these external symbols of success.

These beliefs engender desires in accordance with them rather than in alignment with your Divine Self. If you come from the space of lack, from not having, or from being incomplete, then chasing these desires will result in pain. A belief in separation ultimately manifests the pain of separation.

When you surrender your smaller ego will to your greater Divine Will, you make the intention to move away from separation. Traveling the path of discovery, you see how you created pain and limitation in your life by subscribing to beliefs of scarcity and unworthiness.

In taking responsibility for your choices and the creation of the traumas in your life, you begin accepting your own true Divine Creative Power. Nearing the end of the path, you realize the tremendous source of power at the Core of Your Being, your own True Nature.

Thus, you acknowledge and embrace the paradox. In your act of surrender to Source, you may feel as if the power is outside you. Your surrender opens the gate. And in the end, you come to know that the Power of Spirit has always been within you.

Card for the Day

If this card has spiraled into your life, an issue of separation can now be surrendered. It is an auspicious time to "let go and let God," to surrender your pain, lack of direction, hopelessness, and sense of worthlessness to the Divine Creative Source. It is a perfect time to surrender all that is not working well in your life.

Know that in your act of surrender, you create an opening, a space, for the Divine Expansive Truth to enter. You are choosing to step back and away from the constricted sense of limitation and allowing your belief in lack to dissolve.

Imagine yourself on the top of a mountain. You spread your arms wide to the sky and say, "Not my will, Lord, but Thine." Feel your cares dissipate as the power of Spirit fills you.

Meditation

The act of surrender supported by this symbol involves the choice to let go and empty yourself of all your issues and concerns. Having done so, you can fill yourself again with the grace of your own True Nature.

Spend a little time looking at the symbol's form and color. Bring the symbol up to your heart with the symbol facing your body and visualize the gold color of the symbol flowing into your heart. Then, allow the gold light and the symbol's essence to radiate out from your heart to every part of your body that feels constricted.

See the gold light carrying the symbol's essence, entering each block and dissolving it. It is important to take the time to complete this step without rushing through it. Every area of the body that feels blocked represents resistance to surrendering to your Greater Self.

When the blockages feel cleared, silently state, "*I choose to draw on the highest qualities of this symbol ...*" Feel yourself doing this. Then continue, "*I now surrender and let go of all of my personal issues which have been blocking the fulfillment of Thy plan. I choose to be an open vessel for Source and ask Source to fill my Being and all expressions of my life. So be it. And so it is.*"

However you perceive God, visualize and feel that Holy Presence entering and filling you.

Color and Symbol Balancing

Gold, the symbol's primary color, resonates strongly with the Christ frequency on a universal level and within the Divine Core of our Being.

Yellow, the symbol's secondary color, helps to activate and expand the solar plexus chakra. With this expansion, fears and traumas held in the solar plexus can be released easier.

Violet, the symbol's tertiary color, embodies the quality of transmutation, the ability to shift lower frequencies to higher frequencies of spiritual light.

As a facilitator if you feel your friend has a blockage in his/her solar plexus chakra, you could begin projecting the symbol's essence on a current of yellow light. Silently choose that he or she is able to surrender the issues of powerlessness and victimization held in the solar plexus.

Violet light can also be visualized as infusing and dissolving specific blocks in the energy body. Choose that the symbol's frequency is carried on a radiant beam of violet light. Imagine the Violet Ray filling any darkness or energy constriction in the body and transmuting it to light. You might check for energy blocks in the following areas: kidneys where fear is often held, liver where anger can be stored, and intestines where old memories are often tenaciously held.

Complete the energy balancing session with gold light. Choose that the gold light carry the vibration of the symbol and the Christos essence. Visualize all the individual's chakras filled with gold light and see that light radiating out through his/her whole body.

Lastly, imagine a pillar of gold light running up and down his or her spine, with the gold light column extending through the crown of the head up to the Central Sun and with the lower end of the column extending through the tailbone down into the Earth's core. (See *The Sacred Core Visualization*, pages 45-46.)

When your friend feels deeply connected to All-That-Is, suggest he or she surrender to Source; let go and let God handle the details.

CARD #33

I Am in the Holy Presence of Mother/Father God

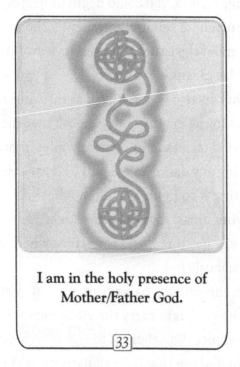

I am in the holy presence of
Mother/Father God.

33

AFFIRMATION

"I Am that I Am."

Insight

This symbol has to do with knowing your true Divine Nature—you are that which you seek. Beneath all the trappings of the personality and worldly beliefs you hold about your identity lies your Divine Core and True Self, the "I Am that I Am." Your Christos aspect is beyond description, words, polarity and conflict. It is also beyond the grasp of your left brain and its approach of categorizing and limiting reality. The Divine and infinite aspect of yourself can't be contained within finite belief systems.

CORRESPONDENCES

PRIMARY COLOR	Gold
SECONDARY COLOR	Purple
TERTIARY COLOR	Silver
METALS\CRYSTALS USED IN GRIDS:	Gold (metal)
	Golden Barite
	Golden Beryl
	Gold Citrine
	Gold Rutilated Quartz
	Sugilite-Luvulite
CHAKRAS CLEARED AND ALIGNED:	Chakras above the head
	Crown Chakra
	Brow Chakra
	Heart Chakra
MERIDIANS CLEARED AND ALIGNED:	Lung Meridian
	Heart Meridian
	Small Intestine Meridian
	Triple Warmer Meridian
PRIMARY ELEMENTS REPRESENTED	
BY THE SYMBOL:	Ether/Fire/Air

The way out of your struggle is through this Divine aspect of yourself. However, to pass through this doorway requires total surrender to the Source of your Being. Like the shaman's little death, the ego-personality's tight grip on your perception is finally seen for what it is and released forever.

From the human perspective, we appear to be a small and rather insignificant piece of the universe. However, each soul is linked through resonance to the entire vibrational essence of the universe. Each soul, like a piece of a holographic negative, holds within itself the knowledge of the whole. We are intimately

"At-One" with the universe, although our third dimensional eyes and ears may convince us otherwise.

The symbol's affirmation, "I am in the Holy Presence of Mother/Father God," alludes to the Divine and Sacred Core within your Being. You are continually in the presence of Prime Creator, and wherever you stand is holy ground. This truth stands against a million beliefs in the world saying it is not so.

This symbol activates the crown chakra and all higher chakras, up to the Great Central Sun. It helps to align you with your Divine Core, resulting in a state of calmness, peace, and tranquility. As you honor your divinity and the divinity in others, the madness of the world fades, the conflict dissolves, and the inherent joy of life returns.

An important aspect of the ascension process is coming to know your own True Nature and accepting fully the Source of your Being. You stop seeing God as separate, in some far distant part of the cosmos, and begin feeling the presence of Source within your heart. In doing so, the full spiritual essence of your Being will seed itself within your body. You can't hold the full spectrum of Light if you continue to feel less than adequate, less than perfect, unequal and insignificant.

When the problems of the world seem excessive, turn within, rather than without, for within is the sacred union for which you search. As holy as you conceive Source to be, so you are! For within you is the spark of Source that you seek, the very fountainhead and essence of your Being. Know that you walk always in the holy presence of Mother/Father God.

Card for the Day

If your Divine Self guided you to this symbol card, your holy presence is being honored. No matter what the world may say, no matter what judgments you or others may have about yourself, know that an aspect of Source speaks, thinks, and acts through you.

The aspect of Source that defines your existence is continually present with you and thus you are always at the throne of Prime Creator. You are connected to the infinite power, wisdom, love, and grace of the universe. You are worthy of this kingdom and nothing less. Cast out all sense of failure, dissolve all feelings of fear and worthlessness. Honor yourself and the Holy Presence you embody.

Meditation

Find a quiet place to rest and meditate. Study the color, shape and form of the symbol. Close your eyes and feel yourself sink deeply into the center of your Being. Silently choose to connect with your Divine Self. When you feel aligned with your Soul Essence bring the symbol card up to your heart (symbol facing your body) and ask, *"Beloved Divine Self, I ask that the purest, highest frequencies of this symbol be transferred to all levels and dimensions of my Being. I now allow myself to fully feel and experience the Holy Presence of Mother/Father God within myself. So be it. And so it is!"*

As you inhale, imagine the gold color of the symbol flowing into your heart and through your entire body. Open your heart and every cell to the gold light. See and feel all fear, criticism, judgment, anger and grief dissolve away in the vibrant presence of the Light. Allow yourself to feel the Holy Presence within you.

Color and Symbol Balancing

Gold, the vibration of the Christ Ray, is the primary color of this symbol. The Gold Ray balances the entire body on all levels and has the ability to transmute "heavy" emotional energies to higher frequencies of light.

Purple, the symbol's secondary color, activates the brow and crown chakras and, being a deeper shade of the Violet Ray, it also carries the ability to transmute blocked energy, allowing it to once again flow freely.

Silver, the tertiary color, resonates with the essence of the Divine Mother and helps balance and equalize the feminine aspect of the body.

The Purple Ray is the first color recommended to be used with the symbol. Visualize and feel the symbol's essence carried on the Purple Ray. See the purple light flowing through the body from the crown to the root, head to foot, flushing out all that is not in alignment with the symbol's frequency.

Follow with the Gold Ray, seeing the symbol's essence carried on a current of brilliant light infusing the body to such a degree it radiates like the sun. Choose that the Gold Christ Ray transmute and clear all that is not like itself. Hold the knowledge, as you do this, that the individual is divine and sacred, as holy as the flame of Source contained within the Core of his/her Being.

If as the facilitator you feel that your friend appears to be ungrounded, I suggest that the Silver Ray be used. Project the symbol's vibration on a stream of silver light, filling the lower chakras (root, sexual, solar plexus) and, if it feels necessary, the left side of the body.

BACK PLATE FOR THE DECK
As Above, So Below

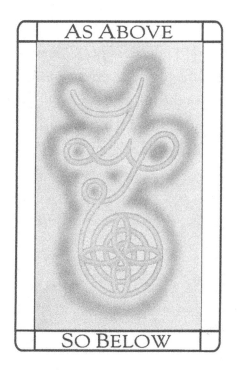

AFFIRMATION

"I call forth the harmonic Waveform of the universe."

Insight

This symbol's essence is about aligning with the Divine Blueprint and manifesting that blueprint on the physical plane.

The holographic expression of the universe allows every part of the universe to embody the knowledge of every other part. Every level of consciousness, even the simplest, such as that of a rock, is linked to the whole, to the Universal Field of Consciousness. Thus, what appears to be "above" is also "below," and what appears to be "without" is also "within."

This symbol represents the unification of dimensions and in turn, an alignment with the highest and most sacred, so that it manifests in our consciousness, in our emotions, and in our physical form.

The symbol titled *"As above, so below"* speaks to the unfolding and flowering of the Divine Blueprint within every aspect of life, and ultimately, to the full expression of Heaven on Earth.

The embodiment of this Divine Blueprint allows for the manifestation of one's Divine Self within our physical body.

Acknowledgements

I wish to acknowledge the following individuals for their encouragement and assistance:

Steven Lord—Steve helped initiate the creation of the Waveform deck by providing the seed money to start the project. He contributed many ideas and suggestions during the composition of the first drafts of the *Waveform Book*. Steve and I spent many hours pooling our intuitive guidance on the most important qualities to emphasize for each symbol. Although I wrote the book, many of Steve's ideas are included in the card descriptions. Thank you, Steve, for helping me take the first step in the grand adventure of creating both the card deck and the *Waveform Symbol Book*.

Paul Bond—Paul was the painter who took my hand drawn *Waveform Symbols* and converted my simple drawings into powerful works of art. The effectiveness of the *Waveform Symbol Cards* can be attributed to his artistic genius.

Jim Vanderhayen—Jim took the digital photographs of Paul Bond's paintings. His skill as a professional photographer played an important role in being able to convert the symbol paintings into the first prototype card deck.

Jai Klarl—The diagrams of human figures in Chapter #3 were drawn by Jai. His artistic renderings definitely improved the quality of the book.

Rick Johnson—Rick supported me with legal and financial

advice, as well as the needed "kick in the pants" when I was losing hope and motivation.

The book's editors, listed in the order of their service:

Pam Cameron—Pam assisted in the first editing of the *Waveform Book*. Pam's skill was deftly applied as she cut away my excess verbiage and guided me in the book's structure and composition.

Joyel Burble—Joyel helped in the proof reading of the book and supplied positive reinforcement during the three years it was being written.

Ruth Sloven—The original manuscript for the book was filed away for years. Because of Ruth's prompting, I resurrected it. Ruth contributed editorial suggestions which were incorporated into the text.

Zhéna—Zhéna proof read the book and caught a number of mistakes that needed to be addressed.

Sally Hanson—I was blessed again with Sally's editorial expertise. She directed me as to the correct punctuation, grammar, word tense and the most appropriate word usage for the book. As always, Sally—thanks.

My Cheering Committee—And thanks to my friends who provided encouragement as I pushed through the writing, editing and re-editing of the book. Your words of support and "pats on the back" helped me find the strength to clear my resistance. Know that you played an important role in the book's creation.

Samuel Welsh

About The Author

Samuel Welsh acquired a B.S. in the Natural Sciences with a focus in ecology. He spent 12 years as a technical writer, writing on subjects such as energy conservation, watershed management, and solar energy. He also wrote operational manuals for electronic equipment.

In 1987, during the Harmonic Convergence, he received a number of spiritual insights which led him to investigate the intangible side of life. He was ordained in the Order of Melchizedek in 1989 and began studying life force energy balancing. He found that his scientific background forced him to constantly develop clear and where possible, rational explanations for his intuitive energetic experiences.

Since the late 1980s he has received certification in the following life force balancing processes: Reiki/Seichim/Sekhem, Frequencies of Brilliance, Esoteric Healing, Soul Recognition, Multidimensional Healing, and Mari-El.

He also utilizes Polarity Therapy (developed by Dr. Stone), flower essence balancing, Matrix Energetics, and two modalities he has created: Multilevel Balancing, and the Polarity Resolution Process (P.R.P.).

Samuel has written three books:

- *Creating Sacred Spaces for Communities: Through Sacred Ratios, Forms, and Placements, Vol. I.*

- *Transforming Inner Stress, The Polarity Resolution Process (P.R.P.), a step-by-step description of the P.R.P. for therapists, counselors, and anyone who wishes to improve his or her health.*

- *The Multilevel Balancing Process, A Life Force Balancing Modality to Assist the Critically Ill and to Support Anyone Who Wishes to Maintain His or Her Health.*

Samuel has provided spiritual counseling and life force energy balancing since 1990. He offers classes and workshops on the following subjects:

- Multilevel Balancing Process—The theory and application of the Multilevel Balancing Process.

- The Polarity Resolution Process (P.R.P.)—How to facilitate a P.R.P. session for an individual, two people in a relationship, and for yourself.

- The Transformational Art of Healing I, II, III—Beginning, intermediate, and advanced techniques of life force balancing.

- Energetic Space Clearing—Ways of clearing and transmuting negative emotional frequencies from land, homes, and property.

- The Waveform Workshop—How to use the *Waveform Symbol* Card Deck to energetically balance yourself and others, to manifest intentions, and to create an energy space for your projects.

- The Basics of Color Therapy—How to use colors to open, clear, and balance the seven major chakras, which in turn support health.

Samuel co-created with the composer/musician Richard Shulman two musical CDs with spiritual frequencies encoded in the music:

- *Ascension Harmonics: Spiritual Attunements through Music.*
- *Keeper of the Holy Grail: Spiritual Attunements through Music.*

(For more information, Search the Web for: "Richheart Music.")

Samuel also helped to produce a sound recording that is free to download from the web called "Tonal Prayers for Mother Earth." This recording helps balance the chakras, meridians, and Earthquake fault lines. (For more information, go to www.tonalprayersformotherEarth.com)

The Great Mystery shines through every form.
Perfection is always present.
S.W., June 2013

CPSIA information can be obtained
at www.ICGtesting.com
Printed in the USA
BVHW042000120520
579550BV00009B/260

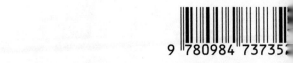